HUNGRY FOR CHANGE
BEYOND THE PALEO DIET

First published in 2022 by Redshank Books

Redshank Books is an imprint of Libri Publishing.

Copyright © Niklas Gustafson

Hardback ISBN: 978-1-912969-31-9

Paperback ISBN: 978-1-912969-32-6

A CIP catalogue record for this book is available from The British Library

Design by Carnegie Book Production

Cover photograph by Oscar Mattsson

Printed in the UK by Halstan

Redshank Books
Brunel House
Volunteer Way
Faringdon
Oxfordshire
SN7 7YR

Tel: +44 (0)845 873 3837

www.redshankbooks.co.uk

HUNGRY FOR CHANGE

BEYOND THE PALEO DIET

NIKLAS GUSTAFSON

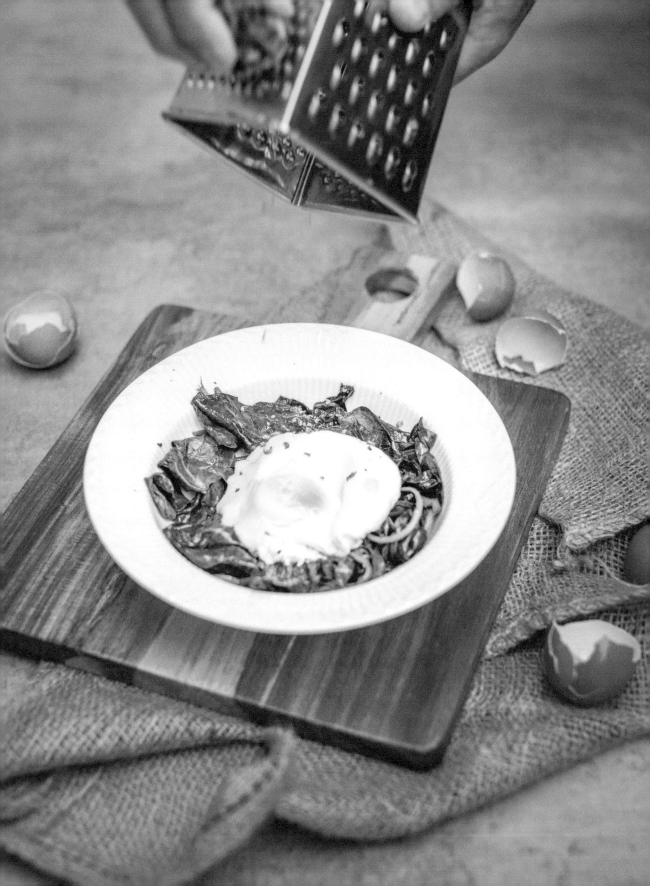

Octavio Laguía

A native of Madrid but a Cantabrian at heart. He studied economics but life took him down a different path, one towards marketing and entrepreneurship. He's a passionate, versatile, and sometimes stubborn guy who is interested in living a natural lifestyle. His greatest loves are his three girls but, he's also fallen in love with living a natural way of life. He enjoys photography and new technologies on his free time. Eating a natural diet has become a fundamental pillar in his personal life and an important project throughout his career. He dreams of a world where the food industry services the health of all and not the pockets of a few. If you ask his friends, they might even tell you that this is an obsession of his rather than just a professional project, which is well reflected in this book.

COLLABORATORS

Oscar Mattsson

A renowned photographer with many awards and his own gallery in his hometown, Gothenburg Sweden. He is passionate about gastronomy and all things food.

Viggo, Lukas and Louis Gustafson

My sons who helped me write this book. They were the best taste-testers and helped me choose the best dishes. :)

Adéle Treschow

Real food enthusiast, her artistic and down-to-earth vision have helped me ground my crazy ideas.

Carmen Ortega

A dietitian and nutritionist as well as a PhD student at Arizona State University (USA).

Gloria Insfrán

Our amazing caregiver and a great friend. She always helps me in the kitchen tirelessly, even when I leave it in complete disarray sometimes.

Laura Ochoa

Food stylist and photographer who greatly contributed to the gastronomic styling you see throughout the book.

Anja Franco Köpke

Journalist and a corporate audiovisual communications specialist with a zeal for gastronomy and literature.

Lorena López

Social media manager and content creator who is licensed in social audiovisual communication and is a fellow foodie.

Lorena Martín

An inquisitive writer with a critical eye for spelling who specialises in project management for online sales.

Sergio Puente
Graphic designer specialising in interface designs and
user experience (UI/UX).

Daniel Sánchez Delgado
Graphic designer, illustrator and food stylist.

Brittany Dubins
American lawyer, writer, and project manager, who was helpful in bringing
this book to life.

Whitney McDavid
A linguist and self-described foodie who is fervent in sharing
cultural idiosyncrasies with others.

As I write this, it's been 14 years since you passed away.

It was too soon. Too soon for us, mom, Jonas, your grandchildren and for me, but especially for you – you, who loved life.

I am convinced that your life did not have to be shortened to only 63 years old if we had known what we know today about nutrition and specifically, the harm of sugar and processed food.

Dad, this book is for you.

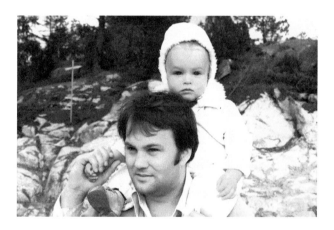

Niklas Gustafson

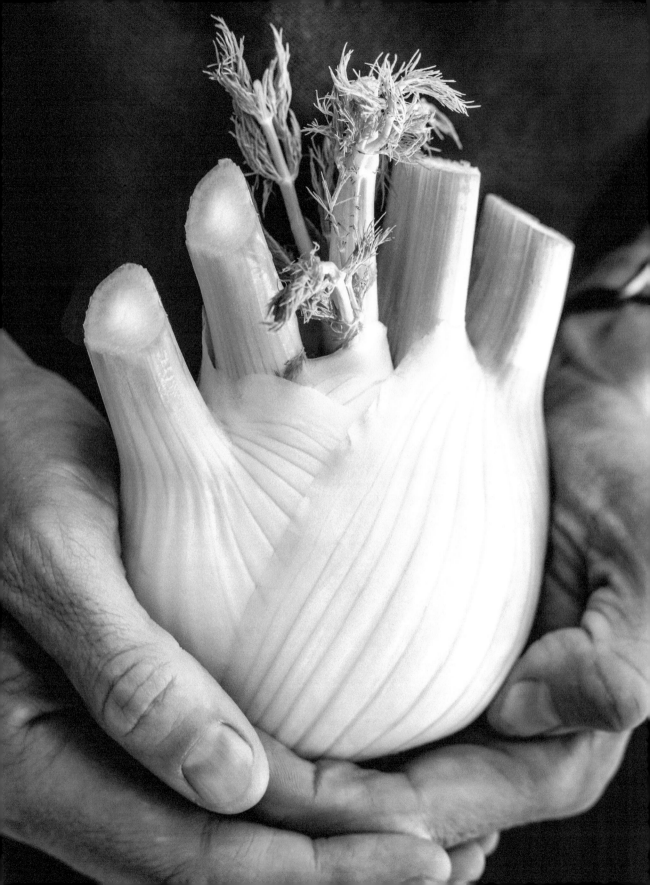

CONTENTS

MY STORY AND THE STORY OF NATRULY...11

THE BUSINESS OF FOOD AND THE TRICKS OF THE FOOD INDUSTRY 25
    Fats: when the good becomes bad 29
    Sugar: when the bad becomes good 36
    A chronological history of deception 44
    Carbohydrates...52
    Other food myths 60

BEYOND THE PALEO DIET...69
    Our origins 73
    The natural evolution of the paleolithic diet 76
    The benefits of a natural diet 82
    Which are the best natural foods? 87
    The importance of exercise 111
    Sleep and rest 116
    The sun and fresh air 121
    Intermittent fasting...124
    Food sustainability 126
    A natural diet for children..128
    Before the recipes 132

RECIPES...135
    Breakfast..137
    Natural smoothies...147
    Appetisers, snacks and breads 157
    Lunch..167
    Dinner...199
    Dessert..229
    Sauces...237

    Recipe index 250

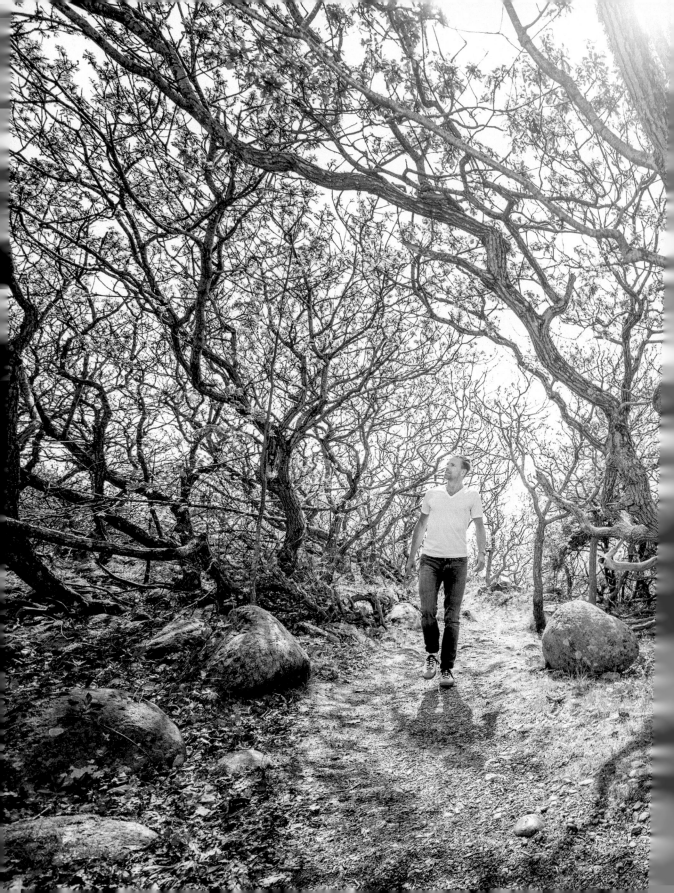

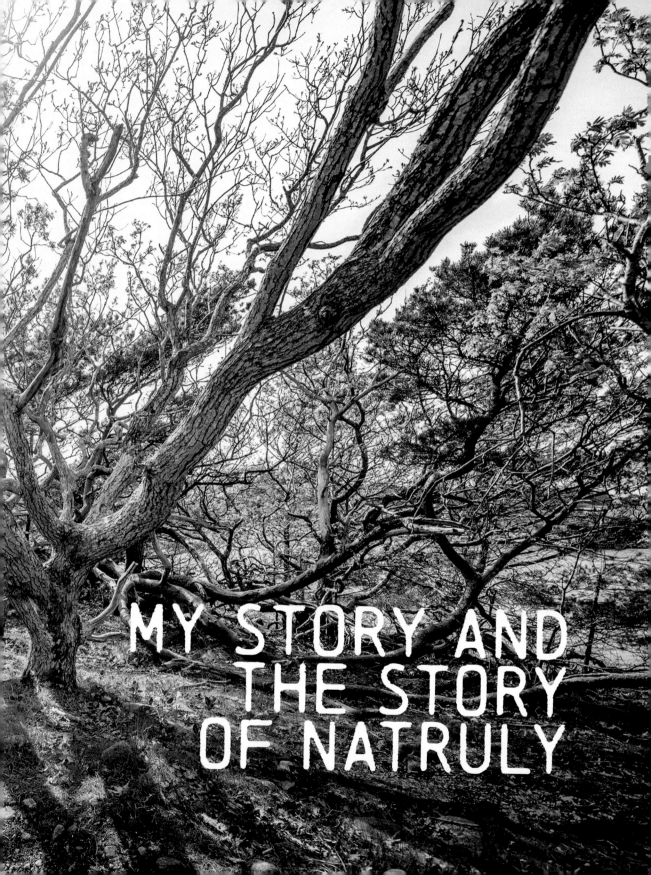

MY STORY AND
THE STORY
OF NATRULY

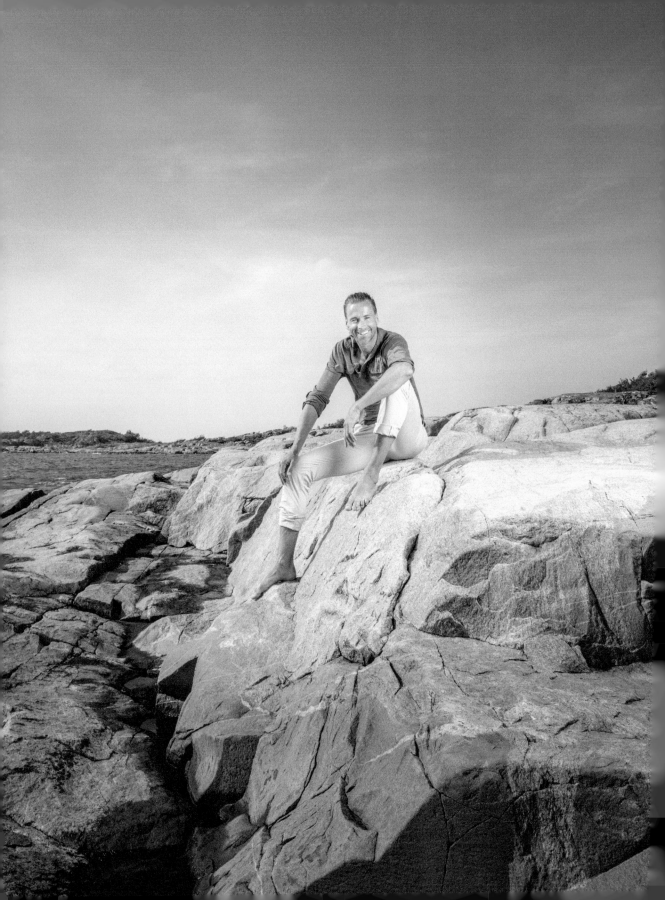

LIKE MOST CHILDREN, I had a happy childhood. A normal, typical Swedish upbringing. I was born in Gothenburg, but we lived in the suburbs outside the city, in a house that was just 2 kilometres from the coast next to the forest. It was truly the best. My brother and I spent hours playing with our friends making tents from sticks we found and with some nails that our parents had given us. We did this almost all year long. We played outside as much as possible, until of course, it got so cold that you could feel it in your bones and the weather made it unbearable. So, as you can imagine we would stop making our tents in the winter, when everything was covered in snow and instead grabbed our sleds and had a blast going up and down the hills over and over again. There is a saying in Sweden – 'there is no such thing as bad weather, just inadequate clothing'.

Near where we lived on the coast of Sweden, it was also very typical to have a small boat. It wasn't anything snobby or elitist actually, quite the contrary. Everyone had some kind of boat, one which they could take out and enjoy going around the archipelagos. Ours was a small one. I hold especially fond memories of it because it's where I spent time fishing with my father and brother. I still remember how easy it was to catch 15 crabs and several lobsters all in one go. In the summer, we had some wonderful family time on the sea as we would sail up and down the Swedish coast for two or three weeks.

Like I said, a typical, happy, Swedish childhood. Although in my case, it wasn't always that way because I was a little different. Before I turned one year old, I began to lose a lot of weight and I was beginning to become more and more malnourished. No one knew what was going on with me, but after months of tests and not getting any better they finally discovered that I suffered from coeliac disease.

In the 70s being coeliac was difficult. There were very few products made for us and the ones that were available were often horrible. I

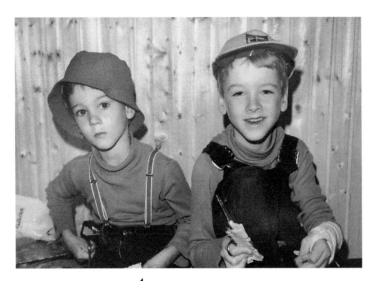

My brother Jonas and I in the sauna painting pictures to sell to our parents' friends, inspired by Picasso and clearly almost identical to his :) 1976

remember that instead of bread they would give me salt-free rice cakes. In fact, they would even spread some margarine on top to make it 'better' (yes, margarine – every time I think about it, I still cringe!) and even with that, they were still disgusting! The worst thing about all of this though was the feeling that I was different. When you're a kid, you just want to be like everyone else. So, when they have to prepare a special cake for you at another kid's birthday party, or a different sandwich on a school field trip... you feel different, you feel less than.

When I was thirteen years old, I became so fed up with the whole situation that I started to eat gluten behind my parents' backs. I ate cookies and other things I shouldn't have. Afterwards, of course, I felt horrible and I would get these tummy aches and these spots on my face. Needless to say, I started taking care of myself again and watched what I ate. I must say though that being coeliac did have some advantages. For example, I noticed my strength. I realised I could live perfectly fine without bread, pasta, cookies, and flour. To be honest I learned an important lesson during that time as a young boy, which was how to read labels. I quickly learned what was good for my body and what was bad. I think that this is where my interest in food came from. Well, that and from both my grand-mothers' kitchens.

MY GRANDMOTHERS AND THEIR PASSION FOR COOKING

When I was a child, my parents often worked a lot and in Sweden, it wasn't common to have a nanny or use a babysitter. Instead, children stayed with their grandparents. So of course, that is exactly what I did. I spent a lot of time with them every day after school.

I loved spending the afternoons with my maternal grandmother and watching her cook the most exotic dishes in her kitchen. My maternal grandmother was born in Kiruna a town in northern Sweden. My grandfather worked in a bank as the head of foreign exports so after they got married, she had the opportunity to travel around the world where she learned a lot about other cultures, particularly their local cuisine. After every trip, she would always bring back some kind of little souvenir but the greatest of them all were the cookbooks and books on spices. This is how she became an expert in exotic cuisine. Her favourite dishes to make were Chinese and Lebanese.

After spending a few days with her it was great to then go and see my paternal grandparents. It was fascinating to see the difference between Swedish cuisine from the north and south. There are a lot of differences between the two. Although, I must say that there aren't as many differences as you would find in a country like Spain, where there is a very rich food culture. In the north of Sweden, they eat things like reindeer, elk, and trout. However, if

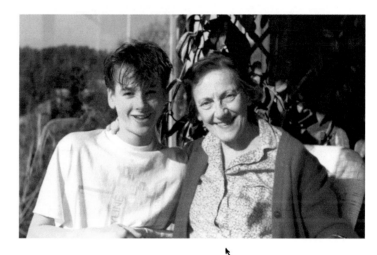

Me, with my maternal grandmother 1982

you are from the southeast of the country like my paternal grand-mother you would eat more seafood and fish. Food from the south of Sweden is more versatile and similar to that of Denmark and Germany. I will never forget the wonderful meals we all shared at my grandparents' table surrounded by family.

I was definitely lucky to have been able to share and enjoy both of my grandmothers' passions for cooking and to have learned and seen all of the different ways there are to cook. By the time I was around 7 or 8 I was hooked! I would go home and spend my time in the kitchen, just learning how to make my own dishes. I started with what seemed like the easiest thing to me at the time and that was a traditional French omelette. As time went on though, I ended up trying to cook anything and everything. I emphasise the word 'trying' here because 9 out of 10 times they turned out horribly. Sometimes my mother would even get upset with me for the amount of food I was throwing away. I never grew tired of trying though. I stuck with it until I got it right. I learned so much by doing

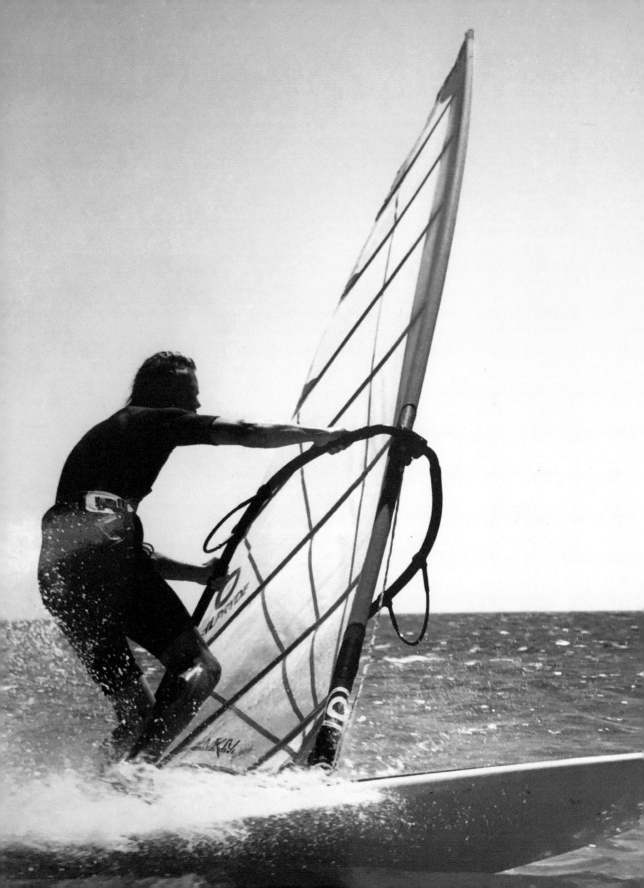

that, the experience was invaluable. Now that I think about it, I realise that I'm not someone who knows how to throw in the towel, it just isn't in my nature. Once I conquered a dish I quickly moved on to the next. I think all of this is burned into my memory because, to this day, I still cook almost daily. It relaxes me, even when it's just for me. I'm always trying new things and I don't stop until I get what I'm looking for, that perfect formula. Another thing about me is that I never cook the same recipe twice. I always have to modify it in some way. If I don't I get a bit bored and feel like it's too monotone. Surely, this is just another thing I got from my grandmothers.

SPAIN AND WHAT I INHERITED FROM MY PARENTS

Another important and defining moment in my life was when I took a year sabbatical. In Sweden, after high school, it's very common for students to take a year off to learn about a new culture and learn a new language. If you could work, it was even better because you showed that you were capable of being independent. Back when I took my sabbatical the normal thing to do was to go to the United States or England – however, I chose Spain. I worked for my friend's father's construction company in Torrevieja selling homes to foreigners and I fell in love with the country. I fell in love with the people, the food, the beaches, the weather, everything really – I could go on and on. At 20, I moved back to Sweden to start my studies at the University of Gothenburg, but I made sure to go back to Spain every chance I got. I did that until I was 28, after which I permanently moved to Spain and started up an internet consulting agency. To this day, I'm still here and working on the various projects that I've created.

> **I chose Spain. I fell in love with the people, the food, the city, the beaches and the weather.**

This entrepreneurial spirit I clearly inherited from my father and paternal grandfather. I'm sure the same is true for many of us when we are children, my father was my brother's and my idol. He was always involved in thousands of business deals, buying and selling everything and he always had new ideas. Looking back now through the eyes of an adult I realise that maybe it isn't the most attractive lifestyle choice, but for us, it is a passion Since we were kids (my brother 4 and I age 6) we put on mini-exhibitions when our parents hosted dinners and other parties where we tried to sell pictures we had painted for a Krona (what would be about 8 pence today). And, by the time we were 7 and 8 we were already going door to door around the neighborhood selling moss we had gathered from the forest to put under the advent candles, a typical tradition in Sweden for Christmas.

We were always thinking about new things to sell so we could earn some money. In fact, when we were 13 and 15, we convinced the manager of our small local tennis club to let us use the storage shed in the garden to sell ice cream, hot dogs and candy during the summer. Our stand became a social meeting point for the club whenever it was open. It was our first commercial success for 3 years (at the level of a 15-year-old, of course).

I inherited so many things from my mother. However, one of them stands out above the rest and that is her interest in new technologies.

My mother is a very cultured woman. She reads a lot and is always interested in the latest things. When I was 15, she put my brother and I in some programming courses (which by the way, no one was doing at the time). They were simple, but she knew it would be useful knowledge in the future. Two years after I started the courses for my 17th birthday my parents gave me a Macintosh SE. This was really the icing on the cake in getting me fully interested in all things related to new technology. At that moment, my mind was made up, I knew I wanted to work abroad doing something related to new technologies.

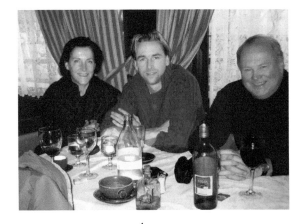

With my parents in Patones de Arriba, 2002

MY FIRST COMPANY AND MY RETURN TO SPAIN

When I was 24 years old, and in my 4th year studying International Business at the University of Gothenburg I got a little tired and just burnt out from studying. So, I decided to set up my first real company, again with my brother by my side along with some other partners this time. I suppose you could say I combined the things I had inherited from both my parents. This was before the boom of the world wide web, web pages and the internet as we know it today. At that time, we developed the graphic design of BBS (bulletin board systems) which at the time were very fashionable and came before the internet forums of today.

We didn't have a lot of technical knowledge, but boy did we want to learn. We visited companies and convinced them that we could do it. In the beginning, it didn't go very well at all. Sometimes it was exasperating as there was little interest in our product. Then, over time and with a lot of hard work we finally started to get traction. We turned our small company into an internet consultancy that got to work for some of the most important Swedish multinational companies.

At 28, I had managed to achieve another one of my professional goals. I sold my stake to a venture capital company in exchange for an investment in the creation of a sister company in Madrid.

So, I took the chance, I packed my bags and came to set up the subsidiary company in Spain.

As I said before, since taking that sabbatical year at the age of 18, Spain had become one of my favourite countries. At 22, I worked as a volunteer for 3 months at the 92 Olympics in Barcelona. At 23, I spent my summer vacation in Tarifa where I fell in love with windsurfing. At 24, I did a study abroad programme in Valencia for 3 months and at 25... I did an internship in Madrid. In 1996, fortunately our internet consultancy agency was doing well, so I was able to continue travelling to Spain several times a year until I finally moved here permanently.

My interest in food composition arose as a result of my intolerance to gluten.

Moving to Spain was an extraordinary experience. The first few years were crazy. I had to set up a new company from scratch but, I always made sure to make time to enjoy and explore everything the country had to offer: its people, its weather, its food and the new passion for windsurfing that I had discovered from my time in Tarifa. I had learned the basics of the sport from my father when I was 10. He had a 'prehistoric' windsurfing board that hardly got used. So, my brother and I would bring it with us on the boat and use it best we could.

However, it wasn't until I went to Tarifa a decade later that I really began to learn how to surf the waves and gain an appreciation for this sport which has turned into a passion.

Up until then my interest in food composition was a result of my gluten intolerance. I inherited my passion for cooking from my grandmothers; my entrepreneurial spirit, from my father, and my curiosity for new technologies, from my mother – and I had discovered my passion for windsurfing in Spain. Spain had given me something else though as well, a zeal for endurance sports.

THE IMPORTANCE OF SPORTS IN MY LIFE

I've always been involved in sports in one way or another. I started playing tennis at a young age; in the winter I skied a lot, like a good Nordic person should. In school I played a lot of different sports too as children do, and at 27 I started running from time to time. Maybe two to four times a month, tops. Nothing serious, but then, 30 hit.

The company that I had started in Spain began to not do so well. I started using running as an outlet, as a way to disconnect. Running made me feel good. It helped me escape from problems and gave me the sense of well-being that I so desperately needed.

To be honest, there was no intention to get healthy on my part. It was out of sheer selfishness. Things weren't going well, and I needed to feel good, it is as simple as that. I needed to go for a run or jog rather, which I did on a gym treadmill. It was just easier at the time, because it didn't matter what the weather was or what the time was, I could just run. I have to say though the thing I liked best about running on the treadmill was that I could see and control my progress in detail (the speed, my endurance), something that wouldn't have been so easy at the time had I been running outside. I ended up running almost every day and training became like a drug for me. It's something that still gives me a sense of peace and happiness without which I couldn't live.

In June 2000 the Öresund bridge was inaugurated, linking the city of Malmö to Copenhagen. It was a huge event in Sweden and Denmark and to mark the celebration they organised a half marathon. My former colleagues from my Swedish company encouraged me to join them in the race.

Of course, I wasn't prepared but nonetheless, the experience was incredible. Almost 80.000 people running together. The feeling you get participating in a race, showing yourself that you can do it, and the fact that you are not competing against anyone but rather with them is just euphoric. The ambiance and type of event itself is unbeatable. From that moment on I was hooked! Back in Madrid, I continued running and I started to participate in other popular races and half marathons, always competing against myself and trying to do better each time. I couldn't stop. My first full marathon was in Madrid at the age of 35 (my friend Johan registered me as a gift for my birthday), so there was no dropping out.

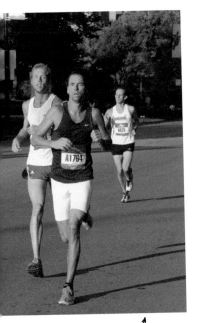

Chicago Marathon 2012

After improving each time over the course of several marathons I was able to get down to 2:46 (my mark in both Amsterdam and Berlin) I decided to participate in my first Ironman at the age of 38, with my friend Luis de Arriba in Austria. I've been in an Ironman every year since.

A TURNING POINT IN MY LIFE

While sports had become a more important and greater thing in my life, the most important change had yet to come. In 2013 a friend of mine told me about a new Paleo restaurant out in Los Angeles, CA. Up until that point I had never of the Paleo diet. She started to tell me about the basics of it and how it was based on what early humans had eaten 2.8 million years ago, primarily cutting out processed foods and sugar. She explained to me that this kind of diet is what made it possible for us to evolve as humans.

My friend had really piqued my interest. My curiosity about food that I had when I was young due to suffering from coeliac disease was reawakened. I also started to connect what she was saying with things my mother had told me about living a healthy life and the war on sugar.

My mother got her taste for healthy living from her mother, my maternal grandmother. She always tried to make sure we ate well. She was one of those people who were ahead of her time. In the 70s she was already convinced that sugar was poison. In fact, she even made sure that my brother and I rarely had any sweets or soft drinks. That is until we turned 10 and 12 years old and started earning money from our little ventures. That's when we started buying ourselves things like candy, ice cream, gummy bears and soda. We would eat healthily overall but, whenever we could get our hands on something sweet, we would take full advantage. It got out of hand pretty quickly. My father was like us in that respect, he would eat sweets all throughout the day, the exact opposite of my mother.

To everyone else it seemed endearing and cute to see always seem him with a sweet in his hand but, not to my mother. So back to 2013, more than thirty years after those first health tips from my mother and grandmother.

While still delving into the Paleo diet and its benefits, I never stopped looking into the food industry and the world of nutrition.

And after some research looking into the Paleo diet, it all started to make sense. Everything I had learned about food and its composition, everything my mother had instilled in me about eating healthily, everything she told us about the negative effects of sugar – everything was starting to come together and make sense. So, I decided to continue reading, studying, and learning about the basics of the Paleo diet.

I read tons of information from as many specialists as I could. Some were from Spain, others from America, northern Europe etc. Some were in favour of it and others were not. Eventually, I began to put the things I was learning into practice. First, by eliminating sugar and afterwards I started to eliminate the few processed foods that I still ate and finally I took the step of cutting out all the restricted foods listed in this diet. It was incredible!

I felt better than I ever had. At 44 I had more energy, felt more focused, and became more active; even my test results during my physical had improved.

It was the straw that broke the camel's back. I decided that I wanted to learn more, seriously learn. I wanted to know everything there was about food and how it affects our body function. So, after two years of studying, in 2016 I got my degree in Dietetics and Nutrition from the University of Cadiz.

As I said before, everything was starting to fall into place. Everything I had learned about nutrition and about the Paleo diet and its health benefits seemed too important to just keep to myself. I had to share it. So, I put all my passions together; my passion for healthy nutrition, cooking, sports and new technology plus my entrepreneurial spirit that I inherited from my father and I launched a blog about the Paleo diet and healthy living. In six months, I had gained more than 60,000 followers. I shared everything I had learned up to that point and showed people that you could eat a Paleo diet while still enjoying tasty recipes that you could make in a fun way.

During that time, I never stopped delving into learning more about the Paleo diet and its benefits. I never stopped looking into the food industry and the world of nutrition because there were many things that did not always sit right with me. There were some commonly accepted concepts that just didn't add up. I thought, 'How is it possible for our society to lead such unhealthy lifestyles?'

That's when I came to the two fundamental realisations that led me to creating my next project with Octavio Laguía: Natruly.

1. First and foremost was the realisation of how the food industry deceives us. It has become a money-making machine where the health of humanity doesn't matter. They don't care if a product is good or bad for our body. They don't care if it hurts us or does us good. Their only goal is to make profits, and huge ones at that.

2. What we want is much more than a simple Paleo diet giving us lists about the foods we should or should not eat. It isn't about strictly following some written rules, it's much more than that. This is about continuing to evolve as a species instead of getting sicker and sicker. This is about leading a natural lifestyle.

Our goal with Natruly is to offer a natural alternative that not only changes how you choose the food you eat, but the way you eat it as well. Today, I'm well aware that what killed my father at just 63 years old was sugar. I'm convinced that his addiction to sugar caused the cancer that took him away from us so soon. And, as I said, although Natruly is much more than a war on sugar, the memory of my father gives me even more reason to continue to fight for the changes I seek.

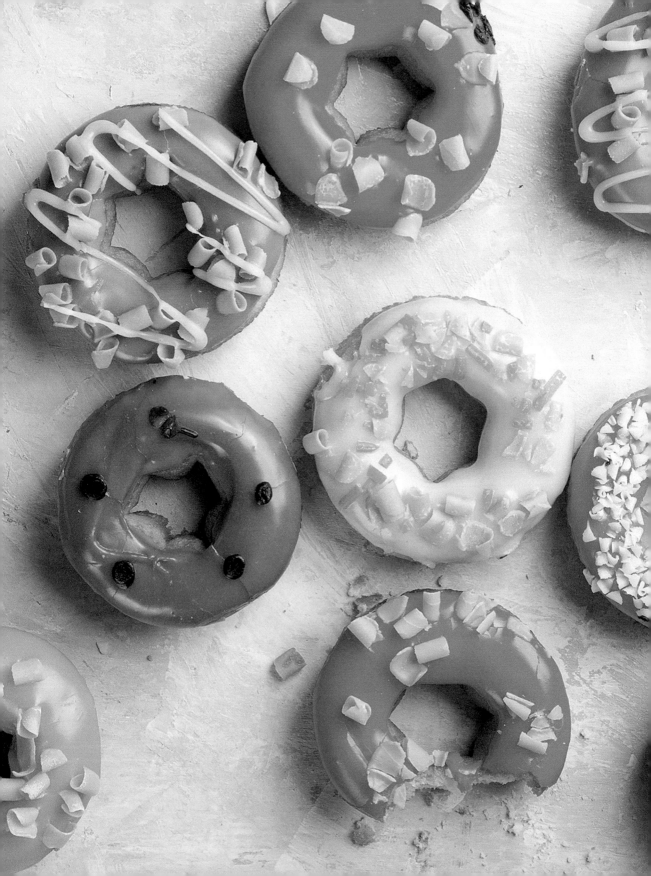

THE BUSINESS OF FOOD AND THE TRICKS OF THE FOOD INDUSTRY

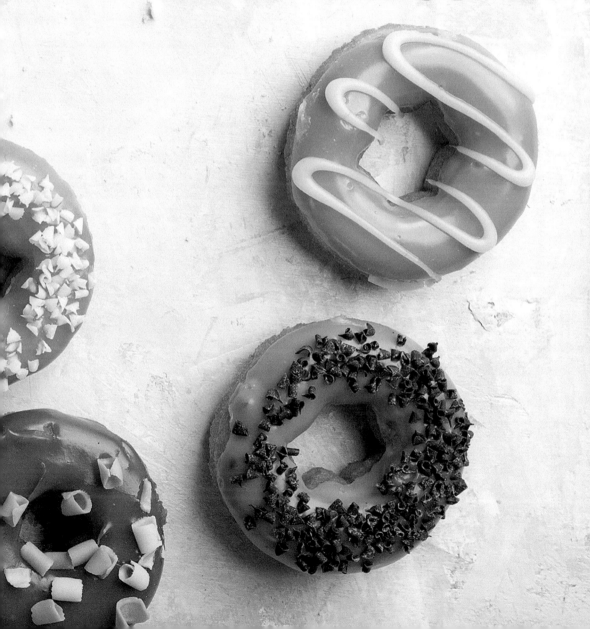

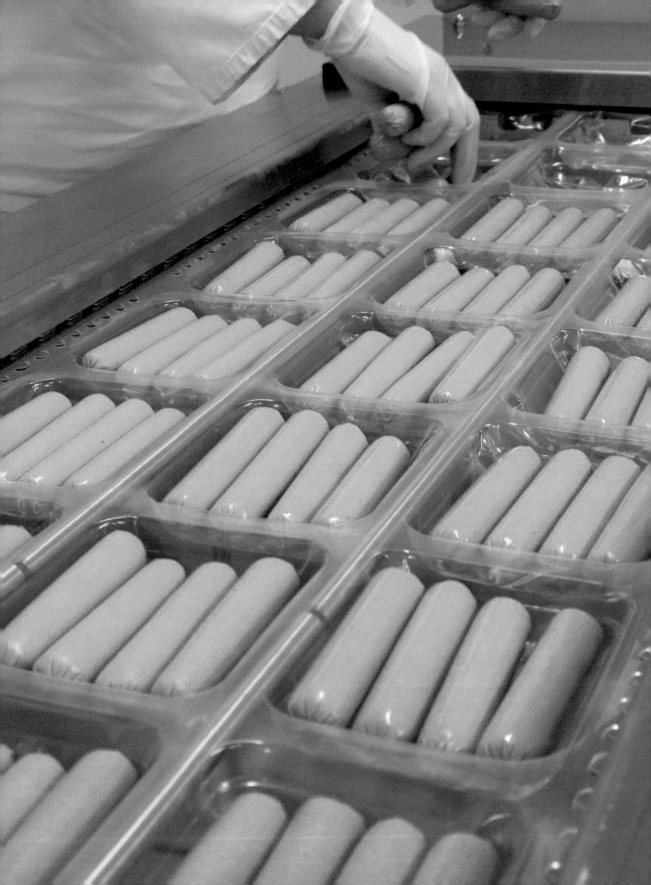

I DON'T KNOW IF THERE IS ANY OFFICIAL STUDY out there or statistical data that supports it, but I am sure that if we ask the first hundred people we see on the street, they would all answer that food is important to them and not just because we need it to 'function'. I'm convinced that those hundred people would say that it is also important for our health. I think the vast majority of people are aware that our health depends greatly on what and how we eat. So, the question is almost obvious: why then do we eat so badly?

The answer however is not so obvious. A lack of time, price, and comfort are some of the most common excuses that we use whenever we ask ourselves this question but, are they really the reasons behind a pattern of eating that has tripled obesity rates since 1970? Are they really the reasons why 41% of children between the ages of 6 and 9 are either overweight or obese? Are they the reason why cardiovascular disease has become the leading cause of death in the UK?

Additionally, if poor diets are directly related to more deaths than, smoking, consuming alcohol and traffic accidents combined; if the majority of cardiovascular diseases and heart attacks could be avoided if we monitored our diet and practised living a healthier lifestyle, then why don't we do things differently? Why aren't we putting more measures into place to implement living a healthier lifestyle?

The answer to all these questions is not that simple. In reality, the answer is hard to accept, maybe even hard to hear, some might even say it sounds paranoid or that I'm being a sensationalist but unfortunately, it is real and can be summed up in one word: self-interest.

That is to say the self-interest of the food industry as a whole. It is one of the most important industrial sectors in the world. Then there is the self-interest of the global pharmaceutical industry which has tripled its profits over the last 15 years, around the world, surpassing the 1 trillion-dollar (US) mark for the first time. Not to mention, the self-interest of the political system where economic contributions from the all-powerful food lobbyist reign high.

The food industry lost its way a long time ago. Food has gone from being a necessity for our health, for our evolution and livelihood to becoming a multi-billion-dollar business where the least important factor is our well-being. A multi-million-dollar business whose main purpose has been to reduce costs, increase benefits and all to the detriment of the quality of our food. A multi-billion-dollar business that has done everything in its power to entice us to consume more and more regardless of the consequences to our personal health. A multi-billion-dollar industry where a few people at the top earn a lot but where the majority of us can and may lose the most important thing in life: our health.

Throughout this chapter, I will discuss some of the biggest scams in the industry from the last few years and how they have had a terrible impact on our bodies.

FATS: WHEN THE GOOD BECOMES BAD

SINCE THE 60s fats have been unfairly persecuted. They've been associated with obesity and cardiovascular disease and have been attacked so viciously that almost everyone in the world associates the word 'fat' with something that is bad and harmful.

Going back to the 1950s, cardiovascular disease – which had barely been present a couple of decades prior – started to become a real public health concern and suspicion began to arise about the excessive consumption of sugar. The food industry, as we'll see later on in our section about sugar, needed a scapegoat to dispel these suspicions and, they found one in fats.

From then on, they started this propaganda machine in order to convince us that excess fat increased cholesterol and that this is what was causing these cardiovascular diseases. And boy did they get it. Top health officials and leading authorities on health all started recommending that we cut out fat from our diet, and we just said, 'ok'. We replaced meat with pasta and rice, butter with margarine, eggs with cereal and whole milk for skimmed milk. In other words, we adopted a diet based on carbohydrates, starches and sugars. The damage was done.

Luckily, all of this started to come to light and some of the scientific community started to acknowledge their mistake. In 2015 the American Medical Association urged the US government to withdraw its recommendations limiting the consumption of fat, and in September 2016, many others including many media outlets, echoed the complaints made by the American Medical Association just a few days earlier (McNamara 2015).

These articles showed with documentation dating back from the last fifty years that what is now the Sugar Association organised a massive and successful public relations campaign against the consumption of fats. They paid renowned scientists and used other tactics so that these scientists would NOT link the consumption of sugar with obesity and cardiovascular disease but rather with the consumption of fats.

Some of these 'paid for' scientists included Dr. Mark Hegsted, the head of Nutrition at the US Department of Agriculture, and, Dr. Fredrick J. Stare, the head of the Department of Nutrition at Harvard and one of America's most influential nutritionists at the time.

Doctor Hegsted, for example, went so far as to use his studies to influence the US government's food recommendations, which pointed to fats as the reason for cardiovascular diseases (O'Connor 2016).

Meanwhile, in the early 1950s, a researcher at the University of Minnesota, by the name of Ancel Keys, who was also funded by the emerging sugar lobby, began to propagate his own idea that fat consumption was directly linked to cardiovascular disease. In just ten years, thanks to his charisma, brilliance, combative spirit, novel theory and support from the right lobbies, Keys was able to obtain institutional power – assuring him and his allies major high-profile positions in important American Health agencies.

Despite all this though, his theory still had critics within the scientific community, as there was no data to support such claims, yet there was data suspecting the disastrous consequences of consuming excessive amounts of sugar.

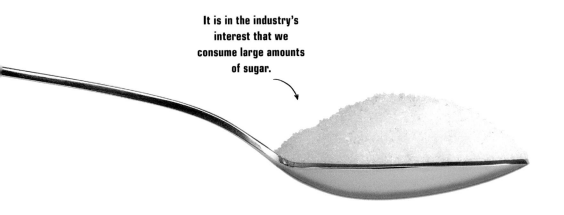

It is in the industry's interest that we consume large amounts of sugar.

So, to combat these critics, Ancel Keys initiated the largest nutritional habits study done up to that point which commonly became known as the 'Seven Countries Study'. Over a few decades Keys analysed more than 12,000 men between the ages of 40 and 59, from seven different countries. This study corroborated Keys' theory (since of course he could have it no other way) that it had been observed that individuals from countries with the highest fat consumption were more likely to suffer from cardiovascular disease. Any opinions opposing or questioning the validity of this study were immediately crushed by the reach, magnitude and forcefulness of Keys (Seven Countries Study n.d.).

Of course, this theory was welcomed by the sugar and refined carbohydrate lobbies. But the reality, and what has been learned in recent years, is that this study was flawed. Some people say that the results were intentionally biased towards the result that was most beneficial for their interests. Others argue that it was simply a misinterpretation of the data. What there is no doubt about today, however, is that the conclusions were incorrect.

The people in charge of our health encouraged us to consume low-fat products regardless of the amount of sugar or carbohydrates

In any case, the word was out and unfortunately, the great success of this marketing campaign led to those in charge of our health to encourage us to consume low-fat products for decades regardless of the amount of sugar or carbohydrates we would eat.

BUT WHY FATS?

Fats were the perfect enemy for several reasons. The first was simple: it wouldn't be difficult to convince people of the association between fats and fat (as fat is already a negative word in the English language). A bit flimsy from a scientific perspective but nonetheless effective, very effective.

The second reason: calories. One gram of fat has twice as many calories as one gram of carbohydrates or protein. Therefore, the relationship between 'more fat, more calories' and 'the more calories the fatter you become' was simple and just as effective.

The third: energy sources. The body's main sources of energy come from fats and carbohydrates. If we eliminate fats we would have to up our intake of carbohydrates, which was of interest to the food industry. Lastly, the fourth, but most important reason: finances.

Among the many necessary properties of fat is its great satiating power. What does that mean? Well, if we consume fat, we are less hungry. The less hungry we are, the less we eat. It is as simple as that. Obviously, that isn't beneficial to the food industry and is therefore something they don't like. So, as a result it was of upmost importance to remove fat out of the equation leaving room for the consumption of other products like refined carbohydrates and sugars.

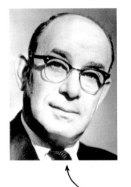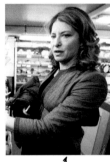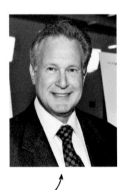

John Yudkin, Nina Teicholz, Robert Lustig

Thus, foods high in fat, especially those high in saturated fat, have been systematically processed to replace fat for refined carbohydrates and sugars, filling our fridges with margarine and yogurts (low in fat, but full of sugar) and filling our pantries with pasta, sliced bread, cereal and cookies. While at the same time demonizing fats. It became the era of low-fat products, refined carbohydrates and all of their variants.

However, there was a spark of hope. In the second half of the 20th century, it was very difficult if not impossible, for opposing voices to be heard in the powerful upper echelons of the industry. Cases like that of Dr. Yudkin, one of the most prominent nutritionists in the UK during the 50s and 60s, who was humiliated and ostracised by all the significant and powerful players who were at the service of the sugar industry. Nevertheless though, in the 21st century, with the evolution of the internet, things began to change. It got harder and harder to silence the critics (aka 'the enemies').

More and more voices were raised against all of this madness and were finally able to be heard. Robert Lustig and Nina Teicholz are two example of people who have been tirelessly denouncing the atrocities committed by the food industry for years and, like Dr. Yudkin, have also been slandered by the industry leaders who, for good or bad, continue to defend the current status quo. Even so, their messages are beginning to permeate the wall that has been built.

Additionally, recent studies, such as the one conducted by the US National Institute of Health – *The Effects of Low-carb and Low-fat Diets: A randomized trial*, published in September 2014 – have shown that a diet low in carbohydrates and rich in vegetables, fats and proteins promotes weight loss and better prevents cardiovascular diseases. It is the latest of more than fifty similar studies to have found this (Bazzano et al. 2014).

Finally, parts of the scientific community have begun to recognise their past mistakes and are stating that they no longer believe that low-fat diets are the answer to helping solve cardiovascular disease, and obesity, but are rather quite the opposite. [Fig. 1].

If fats were removed from the equation, it would mean there would have to be an increase in the consumption of carbs, which was of great economic interest to the food industry.

It makes perfect sense. Obesity and cardiovascular disease started to become a serious problem in the 60s and has only continued to get exponentially worse since then.

Humans have eaten meat, fish and eggs since our origin almost three million years ago. The most natural carbohydrates such as cereals (wheat, rice, corn etc.) and the potato only started to become an important part of our diet around 10,000 years ago when we started to learn and develop how to farm. Sugar, on the other hand, has been gradually incorporated into western diets over the last 300 years. It's been only fifty years since the explosion of sugar consumption in our societies and since the western world made carbohydrates the base of the nutritional pyramid. Also, it has only been during that time that fats have all but practically disappeared from our diet due to their bad reputation.

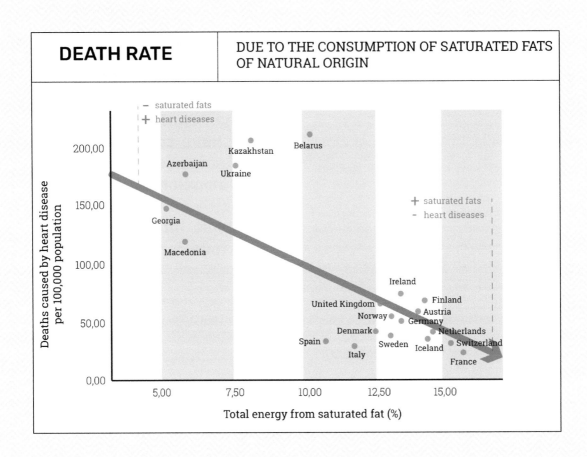

Figure 1: Saturated fats are mainly found in dairy, meats and some oils. Although their consumption, from the 1950s, had been associated with cardiovascular disease, the truth is that countries with the highest consumption rates of saturated fats have fewer deaths from cardiovascular diseases.

They really want us to believe that eating sugar and carbs is NOT linked to increased cardiovascular disease?

Later on, I will explain in greater detail the different types of fats, where they can be found and their qualities and benefits. Right now, though, I'd like to give you some data:

- 50% of the calories from breast milk, the first thing we eat when we are born, comes from fat.

- Fats are vital to the proper functioning of our body. They are essential for our cells and without them many of the vital functions our body must perform, such as absorbing nutrients, would not be able to occur efficiently.

- Fats are one of the most satiating macronutrients. No matter how little we eat, they leave us feeling full for longer, meaning that we don't need to eat in a hurry.

- More and more scientific studies have shown that good fats, such as that from butter, virgin olive oil, or fat from animals that have been fed a natural diet, all reduce the risk of cardiovascular disease.

- Fats boost and enhance flavours. Their presence in a dish makes them more appetising.

SUGAR: WHEN THE BAD BECOMES GOOD

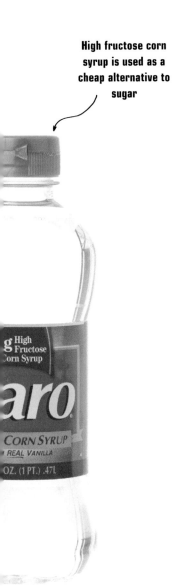

High fructose corn syrup is used as a cheap alternative to sugar

THANKS TO THE INVESTIGATIVE RESEARCH from journalists like Gary Taubes, and the findings of Dr. Cristin Kearns, who found a plethora of historical documents from the sugar industry, and especially thanks to the group of scientists like doctors John Yudkin and Robert Lustig, who have never given up in their fight to show us what sugar really is, a toxic substance that makes us sick little by little. Thanks to people like the ones I've just mentioned we can now shed a little light on the topic. Much of what you will read here is based on their work.

Let's start from the beginning.

WHAT DO WE CONSIDER SUGAR?

By sugar we mean sucrose (the old, granulated sugar, whether it be white or brown) and high fructose corn syrup (HFCS) which is found in more than 74% of the food industry's products, whether they be food or drinks. It has more than 60 names (glucose, fructose, corn syrup, corn sugar, high fructose corn syrup etc.).

High fructose corn syrup was invented in Japan in the late 1960s. It was a cheap alternative to sugar and, at some point in the late 1980s, the American food industry quickly began replacing sugar with HFCS. They peddled the idea that it was a much healthier substance than sugar.

In reality though, sucrose and HFCS are very similar in both their composition and in their harmful effects on our health.

Sucrose is made up of 50% glucose and 50% fructose, and HFCS is a derivative of corn syrup –glucose, at the end of the day – which is processed to add fructose to it in order to get 55% fructose and 45% glucose.

Fructose is actually what gives food its sweet taste. The more fructose there is, the sweeter the food. This is what differentiates sugar from other carbohydrates (which are also sugars due to their presence of glucose) such as breads, potatoes, or rice. They don't contain any fructose but they do contain glucose.

THE DANGERS OF FRUCTOSE

Glucose is such a vital nutrient to our body that if we don't get it through our diet, through carbohydrates, then the body creates it by converting fat or protein through a process called gluconeogenesis.

That is why people like the Inuit (indigenous people who inhabit artic regions like Alaska, Canada and Greenland) have certain levels of glucose in their blood despite having hardly any carbohydrates in their diet. So, although it is a necessary nutrient for life, it is not essential to consume it directly to live. Fructose is another story entirely.

Doctor Robert Lustig, a specialist in paediatric hormonal disorders and an expert in childhood obesity at the University of California's School of Medicine, has spent years researching the effects of sugar and at a conference in March 2016, for the Haas Institute at Berkeley, he presented several studies in which he showed the toxicity of sugar due to fructose (Lustig 2012).

His reasonings were as follows. Fructose is seven times more likely to cause the ageing of cells compared to glucose. Like ethanol in alcoholic beverages, fructose is not essential for life: there is no biochemical reaction in the body that requires it. It does not provide us with any nutrients. If consumed in excess, it is toxic and can become addictive as it stimulates our brain's reward system, thus prompting us to want more and more.

Fructose is seven times more likely to produce the ageing of cells than glucose.

In order to explain why fructose is toxic to the body, Dr. Lustig compared how our body metabolises alcohol and sugar. For example, when we take a shot of alcohol, 80% of it goes to the liver, directly to our mitochondria, which then becomes overwhelmed and is unable to burn it quickly enough. Because of this, it is then expelled through various reactions in the form of new fat that lodges around the liver and as a result creates a fatty liver due to alcohol consumption.

So, what happens when we eat fructose then?

Both alcohol and fructose turn into fat that lodges around the liver.

Imagine we drink a glass of orange juice, which is half glucose and half fructose, or a glass of soda (Coca-Cola, Fanta etc.) which is all glucose. It is metabolised by our body, either in the form of energy or as abdominal or subcutaneous fat due to the unused energy that is leftover. Which is not very pleasant. And, it is ugly.

As with alcohol, all that fructose ends up in the liver and goes straight to our mitochondria which then becomes overwhelmed and cannot deal with all that fructose, so you can't metabolise it. It then gets expelled in the same way as alcohol, in the form of liver fat. Although, in this case, non-alcoholic liver fat, and it is a problem.

It makes so much sense that alcohol and sugar would behave in such a similar way, since alcohol comes from the fermentation of fruit. In fact, the difference between alcohol and sugar is that with alcohol the yeast is what creates the first fermentation process. While with fructose, we are doing that as we consume it. However, once it reaches the mitochondria it doesn't matter where the substance comes from. The damage is the same.

BUT, WHY IS HAVING A FATTY LIVER A PROBLEM?

Over the last 50 years, the specialised scientific community has accepted that one of the major factors, if not the greatest, of having cardiovascular disease and/or diabetes is what is known as metabolic syndrome – despite the media still blaming cholesterol.

According to various studies, having metabolic syndrome means that you are insulin-resistant, which is to say that your cells are actively ignoring this hormone. According to Dr. Lustig's research this resistance to insulin leads to a fatty liver.

SO HOW DOES INSULIN RESISTANCE CAUSE DIABETES OR CARDIOVASCULAR DISEASES?

When we eat, our blood glucose levels rise, especially when we eat carbohydrates. Insulin is then released by our pancreas to help offset these high levels of glucose in our blood stream, it either converts it into energy or, if we have an excess, it will turn it into visceral or subcutaneous fat; you know the type that gives us those love handles that are so difficult to get rid of.

So, if we are resistant to insulin our pancreas reacts by releasing even more insulin in order to try and lower our blood glucose levels. However, if our blood glucose levels remain out of control no matter how hard our pancreas tries to lower them, then our risk of suffering from diabetes is dramatically increased.

On the other hand, if the pancreas continues to release more and more insulin in an effort to overcome your cells' resistance to it, it will at the same time need to generate even higher levels of triglycerides, which leads to higher blood pressure and lower levels of good cholesterol (HDL) and it just becomes a vicious circle and further increases your resistance to insulin. Which in turn, puts you at a very high risk of suffering from cardiovascular diseases.

The conclusion seems clear: the amount of sugar that we currently consume causes fat around our liver, thus making us insulin resistant, leading us to have metabolic syndrome, which then vastly increases the risk of suffering from cardiovascular diseases, diabetes and obesity. This doesn't happen overnight of course, but rather slowly. However, needless to say, it doesn't make it any less dangerous.

Many recent studies have shown the relationship between liver fat and cardiovascular diseases and type 2 diabetes.

Robert Lustig himself, along with his team, conducted a study in 2016 with forty-three obese adolescents to assess how a reduction of sugar in their diet would affect their health (Lustig 2016). They did this in a very special way; they completely cut out sugar from their diet for ten days. On top of that, in order to avoid a hypothetical improvement due to a loss of weight, none of the candidates were allowed to lose any weight.

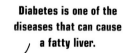

Diabetes is one of the diseases that can cause a fatty liver.

To do this they substituted the calories from sugar to that of starches with things like potatoes, breads etc. The results were overwhelming. In just ten days both blood pressure and blood sugar levels lowered by 5%. Insulin levels lowered by 25%, triglycerides by 46% and liver fat by 22%. All of this was done without losing a single gram.

Nonetheless, Dr. Lustig recalls the defence that sugar advocates have always used, stating that all substances are harmful when consumed in excess. Therefore, sugar is no different and should not be criminalised. For example, Vitamins A and D as well as iron can be harmful when taken in excess. Even too much oxygen or water could harm us and even cause death, but none of those are considered to be toxic substances. Which is true. The big difference though is that just like alcohol or drugs, sugar is addictive, making it more likely to be abused, which is what makes it so dangerous.

These days we consume twenty times more sugar than a century ago! It has gone from being something we just added to our coffee here and there to becoming a staple of our diet. Sugar is present in almost every product that the food industry makes.

It could be even worse.

WHAT IF THE INCREASED CONSUMPTION OF SUGAR IS ALSO RESPONSIBLE FOR THE INCREASE IN CANCER CASES?

As Gary Taubes points out in his research published by the *New York Times* in April, 2011, the relationship between obesity, diabetes and cancer was first highlighted in 2004, after several important studies were done by the International Cancer Research Agency, who are associated with the World Health Organization (Taubes 2011).

However, it really seems that the rise in cancer has gone hand in hand with the rise in cardiovascular diseases, obesity and diabetes since the late 19th century.

Most cancer researchers point to our diets and pace of life as the reasons why we have seen an increase in cases. There is no doubt that this is true and that both these factors are also related to obesity, diabetes and metabolic syndrome.

Taubes stated in his article that Craig Thompson, the president of the Sloan-Kettering Memorial Cancer Center in New York explained that the cells, in many human cancers, depend on insulin in order to grow and multiply.

This means that the constant and uncontrolled secretion of insulin favours the growth of tumours. Thompson further believes that many pre-cancerous cells would never mutate into malignant tumours if they were not being stimulated by insulin, taking up more and more blood sugar to metabolise.

Like alcohol or drugs, sugar is addictive, which is what makes it so dangerous: today we consume twenty times more sugar than just a century ago.

On the contrary, Lewis Cantley, director of the Cancer Center at Beth Israel Deaconess, Harvard Medical School, argues that 80% of all human cancers are driven by their mutations or by certain environmental factors that work to mimic the damaging effects of insulin on emerging cancer cells (Science Watch 2010).

Much of the current research on the link between insulin and cancer is focused on finding drugs to suppress insulin signalling in early cancer cells to try and either completely inhibit or prevent their growth.

In short, sugar consumption creates fat in the liver, this fat is then a precursor to metabolic syndrome and insulin resistance. Being insulin-resistant causes us to release even more insulin into our body and according to these latest studies, excess insulin favours the growth and development of cancer cells.

So, how long will it take to reliably show that sugar is linked to cancer?

GOT IT: SUGAR IS BAD. BUT ARE WE REALLY CONSUMING TOO MUCH OF IT?

It may seem obvious that the United States has a serious problem with the nutrition of its population when thinking about obesity and related diseases. But, to what extent is this a 'fat' problem? How much sugar do they consume? And how much do we consume in Europe and in the UK?

The truth is that the data are alarming.

According to the National Health and Nutrition Examination Survey (NHANES) (CDC 2020), 38% of the adult population is obese in the US. The figures in children have tripled since 1980 and currently sit at 18% in obesity. Cardiovascular disease is the leading cause of death, closely followed by cancer. Between the two they add up to 46% of the total. Also, the average sugar consumption, according to data from the Department of Agriculture, reaches 34 kg per person per year.

In general when we think of Europe and the UK, our feeling is that our numbers are lower. However, the data is actually very similar, or even worse. According to the Health Survey for England 2019 (NHS Digital 2019), more than 64% of the total population of England is overweight (36.2%) or obese (28%). What is even more alarming is that in children between the ages of 10 and 11 years old, the percentage of obesity is 21% and of overweight 14.1%. Meanwhile, in Europe, according to Eurostat (Eurostat 2019), the data is very similar: 36% of adults are overweight and 17% are obese. As we can see by these numbers, it is a general misconception that being overweight or obese in Europe is not an issue.

Regarding cardiovascular diseases and cancer, these are also the leading causes of death in Europe, but the data is even worse than in the US: 37% for cardiovascular diseases and 26% for cancer. Between the two diseases they account for more than half of all deaths (Eurostat 2021), and consumption of sugar, according to the Uk's 2020 Sugar Intake Report (Public Health England 2020), is through the roof: 43.4 kg per year per person in the UK and 34 kg in Europe in general.

Just to give you an idea – 34 kg of sugar per year per person consumed in Europe or the US is equivalent to eating 23 teaspoons of sugar a day.

You might be thinking, 'How? That seems impossible. I don't even add sugar to my morning coffee!'

Well that is where the food industry comes into play and every-thing that I have told you thus far about high fructose corn syrup and the many other names that the food industry gives sugar to make us think we are not consuming it. Sugar is almost omnipresent in Western food. As we have already said, sugar is present in 74% of the products of the food industry, so almost certainly every piece of bread you eat, every cookie, every mid-morning snack, every sauce, every piece of pizza, every sausage, every hamburger, every branded meat tray, every dessert, every yogurt, every soft drink, and so on, countless examples bring us closer to that incredible figure.

To put these 34 kg into perspective, it is only necessary to take into account the recommendations of the World Health Organization

(WHO) (and, as you will see a little later, we will have to 'take them with a pinch of salt'). The WHO recommends that we consume below 5% of our daily calories in the form of sugar and urges us to consume no more than 10% (WHO 2015). In other words, the WHO recommends that we try to consume less than 14 kilos of sugar per year. And we are at 34...

HOW IS IT POSSIBLE THEN, WITH SO MUCH EVIDENCE THAT THE USE AND CONSUMPTION OF SUGAR IS NOT MORE REGULATED?

It is incredible, but despite all this evidence and data, most health authorities in every country continue to allow the indiscriminate use of sugar by the food industry. What is even more appalling, is that they allow it to be given to children without even warning people of its consequences.

More and more children are becoming obese, getting fatty livers and being diagnosed with type 2 diabetes. Cardiovascular diseases and cancer are responsible for the majority of deaths Europe. Despite all of this, we do nothing.

Unfortunately, there is a reason why.

We consume a lot of sugar without even realising it.

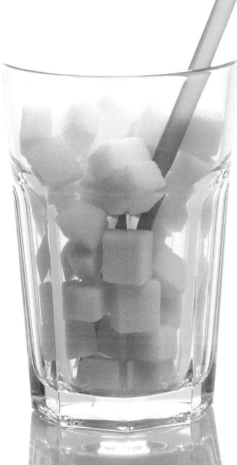

A CHRONOLOGICAL HISTORY OF DECEPTION

AS WE HAVE ALREADY SEEN, despite the amount of evidence that has existed against sugar for decades it has become one of the most widely consumed products. The history of its use and popularity is closely and directly linked to the persecution of fats. And, truthfully its story has everything needed to become one of best scripts in Hollywood. Intrigues, conspiracies, good guys, bad guys, and an unbelievable ending, an ending that looks like it's going to be awful.

The bad part is, it's not a movie, it is reality, and we are the victims. The good part though, is that we still have time to change the ending.

Once again, thanks to the work of Gary Taubes and Cristin Kearns, among others, we can learn about the true story of sugar and the huge media campaign that benefited the industry. I've summarised below, in chronological order, how we got to where we are.

1200
In India, they developed a process to extract the juice from sugar cane and started to make the first sweets. It was extremely expensive and rare, which is why it was only intended for nobility. It is the first record we have of the use of sugar.

1700
The mass production of cane sugar begins, but it remains extremely expensive until the middle of the 19th century.

1900
Sugar consumption is beginning to be suspected as the reason behind an increase in diabetes when compared to societies with little to no presence of sugar in their diet, and whose incidences have remained low.

1924
According to Haven Emerson, director of the Institute of Public Health at the University of Columbia, the cases of diabetes in New York increased 15 times during the same period of time as the increase in sugar consumption

1942

Authorities are beginning to take the issue of excessive sugar consumption seriously. The US government launches a campaign to make people aware of the fact that sugar is not a necessary part of our diets. Sugar consumption in the United States is cut in half, making the total per person per year just 10kg.

1943

The sugar industry is beginning to get concerned about the decline in consumption and creates the Foundation for Research on Sugar, whose mission is to study the positive effects of sugar in your diet. They then publicise their research. The first study on metabolising sugar was commissioned by Ancel Keys from the University of Minnesota, he had a budget of 36,000 dollars (which is equivalent to 500,000 dollars today).

1952

During the Korean War, pathologists who performed autopsies on American soldiers killed in combat found that many had a significant level of platelets in their arteries, unlike their Korean counterparts (Ahrens et al. 1957). The difference was attributed to the fact that Americans had high-fat diets, where the Koreans did not. What was not indicated is that Americans had a diet that was rich in sugar, where the Koreans did not.

1953

Campaigns begin, advertising sugar as the healthier 'food' and turning it into the perfect ally for staying thin.

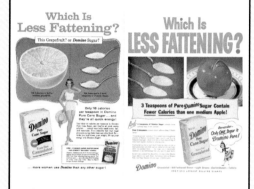

1955

US president Eisenhower has a heart attack which puts cardiovascular disease on the front page across the world. A race against the clock begins to search for the cause that is increasing these kinds of ailments.

1956

Ancel Keys, the first researcher funded by the sugar industry, begins a massive study to find the cause behind cardiovascular disease. It is known as the 'Seven Countries Study'.

1958

Ancel Keys starts to spread his theory that fats are the reason for the increase in cardiovascular diseases.

1960	

John Yudkin, the UK's leading nutritionist at the time, begins a series of experiments and research to better understand the effects of sugar consumption in both humans and animals.

1961	

Thanks to his great personality, his natural gift of relating to people and for having the right contacts, Ancel Keys becomes a relevant and popular figure both in and out of the scientific community.

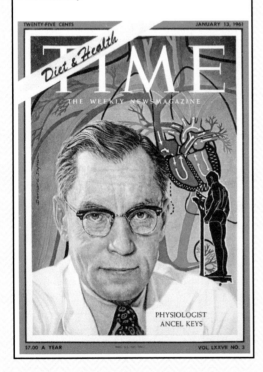

1970	

Ancel Keys publishes the first results of his monumental study, on over 12,000 subjects, which was financed by the American Sugar Lobby. The 'Seven Countries Study' directly linked high-fat diets to cardiovascular disease. But, as we saw in the chapter on fats, the study was biased.

1971	

Keys publishes an article directly attacking Yudkin and calling his anti-sugar studies 'flimsy'. He attacked him with such vigour and contempt that Yudkin was never able to recover in the eyes of the media.

1972	

Despite everything, Yudkin publishes his controversial book *Sweet and Dangerous* (Yudkin 1972) and his book *Pure, White and Deadly* (Yudkin 1972), where he presents the conclusions from his studies. In them, he points out that sugar increases the level of triglycerides in the blood, which, both then and now is considered to be one of the greatest risk factors for cardiovascular diseases. He also argues that it raises the level of insulin which is directly related to type 2 diabetes. Almost no one in the scientific community at the time paid attention to Yudkin's studies due to the 'bad press' he had received years prior for his opposition to sugar and low-fat diets.

1973	

The United States Department of Agriculture becomes suspicious of sugar thanks to the research done by Doctor Sheldon Reiser and Doctor Judith Hallsfrich (Reiser et al. 1973).

1975	

The Sugar Association, concerned about the new and emerging doubts related to sugar, decides to hire the public relations firm Carl Byoir & Associates to quell these doubts. Their first action is to publish a fresh paper called Sugar in the Human Diet, edited by Dr. Frederick Stare, founder of the Department of Nutrition at the Harvard School of Public Health. The paper offered a set of arguments in favour of sugar which could then be used against its opponents. 25,000 copies were distributed to journalists with a press release that said: 'Scientists dispel fears about sugar' (Stare 1975).

1975	

The sugar industry runs newspaper and magazine ads promoting their product as a healthier nutrient: 'Sugar can be the willpower you need to eat less'.

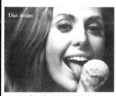 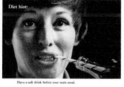

Sugar can be the willpower you need to undereat.

Sugar just might be the willpower you need to curb your appetite.

1975	

Attacks on Yudkin reach their peak. Keys publicly labels Yudkin's research propaganda and calls his findings simply wrong.

1975	

Frederick Stare, mentioned above, becomes a spokesperson for the Sugar Association and appears on various media platforms advocating for the consumption of sugar in our diet.

1976	

Given the debate that was being generated in American society, the FDA (Food and Drug Administration) had no choice but to review the effects of sugar on our health. They commissioned a study from the Federation of American Biological Societies Experiment, which created an expert committee led by George W. Irving Jr. Coincidentally, Irving had recently been head of the sugar lobby's expert committee. Of course, this committee then concluded that it did not find credible or reasonable evidence of biochemical damages resulting from the consumption of sugar. We now know that six of the fourteen studies used to reach such a conclusion were commissioned by the Sugar Association. Based on the conclusions presented, the FDA included sugar on the American list of Generally Recognized as Safe (GRAS) for consumption. From that moment on the food industry had the power to use as much sugar as it wanted in their products (Taubes 2016).

1976

The sugar industry launches a new ad campaign, taking advantage of the 'good press' they are receiving. There were many ads, but one that stood out was 'Sugar is safe! It does not cause death or disease... The next time you hear someone knocking on sugar, watch out for their lies'!

1976

Dr. Frederick Stare's conflict of interest with the sugar industry becomes known, however his propaganda work has already been spread around and the Sugar Association no longer needs his services.

1976

John Tatem Jr. and Jack O'Connell Jr., president and director, of public relations for the Sugar Association receive the Silver Anvil award (the Oscar of the public relations world) for their excellent work in 'shaping public opinion' – incredible but true.

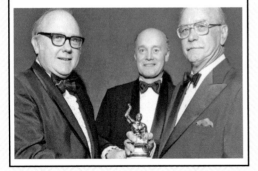

1980

The US Department of Agriculture publishes its first dietary guide based on the writings of Dr. Bierman, a nutritionist at the University of Washington and a panellist hired by the Sugar Association. The guide states, 'contrary to what many people believed, consuming large amounts of sugar does not seem to cause diabetes'.

1980

With sugar off the hook, low-fat diets start taking the world by storm and become part of societies' everyday diet. Obesity in the US continues to rise and affects 14% of the population.

1984

Time magazine publishes an attack on fat with the cover of their magazine (*Time* 1984). Obesity, diabetes, and cardiovascular diseases continue to rise as sugar consumption in the US reaches 34kg per person per year.

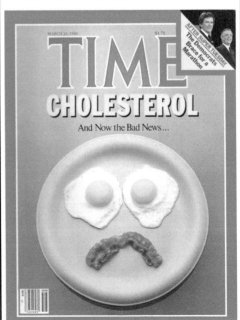

1985

While the US Department of Agriculture's Laboratory for Nutrition and Carbohydrates (USDA) warns that even low amounts of sugar intake might be contributing to cardiovascular disease, the USDA itself updates its dietary guide and, keeps the 1980 recommendation which stated: 'eating too much sugar does not cause diabetes'. This was done by Dr. Frederick Stare a former spokesman for the Sugar Association.

1986

The FDA publishes a report that points out that there is not a concise agreement within the scientific community regarding the amount of sugar intake that is suitable for human consumption. This report seemed to exonerate sugar for problems such as obesity, diabetes, and cardiovascular disease (New York Times 1986).

1995

John Yudkin, the leader on the fight against sugar, dies. The soft and sugary drink industry is now already producing enough for each person to consume 200 litres per year!

2000

Sugar-related diseases are skyrocketing. Sugar consumption in the Unites States reaches 54 kg per person per year. The percentage of people who are obese worldwide reaches 16% with the United States standing at 33% of all people being obese.

2002

Gary Taubes, an independent researcher at the Robert Wood Johnson Foundation, reopens the debate on sugar in his article published in the *New York Times*, 'What if it's all been a big fat lie'? In the article he uncovers some of the practices used by the sugar industry and looks into the studies they carried out (Taubes 2002).

2003

The World Health Organization for the first time, recommends that sugar consumption should not exceed 10% of our total caloric intake. Andrew Briscoe, president of the Sugar Association wrote a letter to the CEO of WHO saying that the association 'would take every available avenue to them to expose the dubious nature of their reports and would urge the committees responsible for congressional budgets to reconsider future funding to the WHO'. Additionally, the Association approached then United States Secretary of Health and Human Services, Tommy Thompson, requesting his 'prompt and favourable attention' regarding the official publication of the WHO's report. Thompson's team responded with a letter detailing that 'the policy recommendations and interpretation of science of the US government differ with those stated in the report from the World Health Organization'. After that WHO did not follow through with their recommendation.

2005

The United States Institute of Medicine publishes a report similar to the one written by the FDA in 1986 concluding that 'there is a lack of consensus in the scientific community regarding the amount of sugar intake that is recommended for a healthy diet'.

2009

Three decades after Dr. Yudkin's research, Dr. Robert Lustig gives a speech where he again links sugar to cardiovascular diseases and type 2 diabetes. The video reaches more than 7 million views on YouTube.

2010

The USDA updates its dietary guide again, however this time it is based on the reviews from nutritionist Sigrid Gibson, who worked for the Sugar Bureau and the World Sugar Research Organization, and from Carrie Ruxton, the former head of research at the Sugar Bureau until 2000. The guide still states that sugary drinks are not fattening.

2011

The United Nations reports for the first time in human history that non-infectious diseases such as cancer, cardiovascular disease and diabetes pose a greater threat to global health than infectious diseases. They point directly to the consumption of alcohol, tobacco and a poor diet as responsible for the rise in non-infectious diseases. Tobacco and alcohol are regulated, but what about products related to our diet?

2012

Doctor Cristin Kearns discovers secret documents from the sugar industry which reveal the lies and deceptions they have used in their massive public relations campaigns since the 1970s. Kearns contacts Gary Taubes and together they publish the truth about everything and expose the inner goings-on at the Sugar Association in the magazine, *Mother Jones* (Taubes 2012).

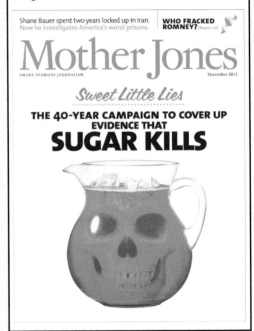

2014

Mexican Authorities, in a clear fight against obesity rates, approve the first ever tax against soft drinks despite the objections from companies making processed foods. Sales fell 12% the following year.

2014	

An influential study published by the *Journal of the American Medical Association* (JAMA) links the consumption of sugar with the risk of mortality from cardiovascular disease. This comes 40 years after Yudkin and Reiser first concluded that. Finally, it seems like the world is listening (Yang et al. 2014).

2015	

Doctor Cristin Kearns continues to delve into the documents she uncovered about the Sugar Association. She publishes her first report against the sugar industry. Her findings have an international impact. People are ready to transform the sugar industry in the way the tobacco industry has already been transformed.

2015	

The World Health Organization finally publishes an official guide on sugar consumption. It recommends for sugar never to exceed 10% of our total caloric intake, although it says it is preferable to remain under 5%. This translates into no more than 18kg per person per year but with a recommended 9kg per adult per year (WHO 2015).

2016	

According to WHO the number of obese people is 30% higher in wealthier populations compared to that of poorer populations.

2018	

More than 50% of adults in member countries of the OECD (Organization for Economic Cooperation and Development) are obese. It is estimated that there are more than 2.2 million people who are overweight around the world.

As we just saw, this is the story of one of the largest and most efficient marketing campaigns in history. One that has had clear winners (the food industry) and clear losers (the people). A campaign that not only put the food industry in the spotlight, but also our health authorities and governments, who thought more about their personal interests rather than those of the entire population that they swore to protect.

With that said, there is still something encouraging about this timeline, something that we can lean on to be hopeful and optimistic, and that is what has happened over these past few years. More and more voices have risen against this food pyramid model that has been pushed upon us, and more and more official organizations such as the WHO, are wanting to take this seriously. There is still a lot that needs to be done, but we are starting to see the light at the end of the tunnel.

CARBOHYDRATES

NOW THAT WE HAVE SEEN WHY and how sugar hurts us, and how the food industry has taken advantage of their position over the last fifty years by disproportionately increasing consumption of their products to continue to increase their profits, let's take a further look into what they are currently doing.

In recent decades another ingredient has been pushed upon us, which we might want to reconsider: carbohydrates. Most rice potatoes and cereals – especially wheat, which is used to make flour, bread, pasta, pizza etc., have been modified over the years so that we have to eat larger and larger amounts of these foods to stay feeling 'full'. We have designed these foods to our liking, but as a consequence of these modifications such foods have lost their nutritional value and actually give us very little.

But to better understand how carbohydrates affect us and what they actually provide us, we must take a small step back.

Pasta makes us feel full, but it doesn't nourish us. It should not be the basis of our diet!

TYPES OF CARBOHYDRATES

Carbohydrates are found in nature in two forms:

- **Simple Carbohydrates** these names refer to their chemical structure. Simple carbohydrates are composed of one or two kinds of sugars. These are quickly absorbed by the body and can be found in cereals, milk, fruit and in some kinds of vegetables.

- **Complex Carbohydrates:** are starches and fibre. Their structure is made up of two or more sugars, generally linked by a chain. They are mostly rich in fibres, vitamins and minerals. Due to their complexity, it takes longer to digest them, which means that they provide us with longer-lasting energy. They are commonly found in tubers, vegetables, and legumes.

And humans have created a third kind:

- **Refined Carbohydrates:** These are either simple or compound carbohydrates that have been processed to consume by stripping them of all their bacteria, bran, nutrients and vitamins. This group includes all industrial foods such as breads, pastas, pastries, sweets, soft drinks, alcoholic beverages – any processed food.

Once we know all of this, we have to take into account other important aspects when assessing macronutrients. Mainly, how they are found.

Carbohydrates can be found in the form of fibre in combination with other micronutrients; they can appear practically on their own, nutritionally speaking, in which case they act as empty calories, and even as part of other foods that also provide us anti-nutrients.

Anti-nutrients are compounds that essentially protect plants, like seeds, cereals and legumes from bacterial infections, and from being eaten by insects. It has been proven though that these compounds interfere with humans' ability to absorb nutrients and after long periods of consumption can cause digestive problems, all kinds of allergies and have even been linked to some other more serious illnesses. Therefore, it is crucial that we properly select where our carbohydrates come from.

Let's go back a step further to have an even better idea or what we are talking about.

WHAT ARE CARBOHYDRATES AND HOW DO THEY WORK

We already know that carbohydrates, together with protein and fats, form the fundamental group of macronutrients that our bodies need, and that their main function is to provide us with energy. However, what we often don't realise is that although there are essential fats and there are essential proteins (amino acids) there are no such essential carbohydrates. If necessary, we could live without carbohydrates, but we couldn't live without fat or protein.

Once we eat carbohydrates, our body releases insulin in order to convert them into glucose, which we then use for energy.

Everyone knows that we need energy to 'function'. Even still, people were able to be convinced over the last half of the 20th century that fat, an even better source of energy for humans, was not good for us.

In the first past of this chapter, you read about why the sugar industry needed to find a culprit for the alarming rise in cardiovascular diseases, obesity and type 2 diabetes and what they chose to blame: fats. This was all to dispel the doubts around sugar and its consumption. The result of their efforts, as you now know, was that since the 60s fats have become public enemy number one. Thus, they were practically eliminated from our diet. Which in turn, clearly helped the sugar industry and paved the way for its increased use. The industry also benefited through something else though: carbohydrates.

If the human body has two main sources of energy, and we get rid of one of them, what happens to the other? Simple, we will just have to overcompensate for the loss of one with the other. This is in short, what happened between fats and carbohydrates. Again, this benefited the food industry as it further increased the development of refined carbohydrates, used in white bread, flour, pasta, pastries etc.

This switch from fat to carbohydrates had a hidden danger. It wasn't just a simple exchange of one type of energy for the other.

Simple and refined carbohydrates, due to their composition, are absorbed rapidly in the body, which means that they immediately cause a high level of sugar to be present in our blood. This forces the pancreas to convert that sugar into energy by releasing a proportional amount of insulin in order for our body to try an metabolise the sugar.

When reasonable amounts are consumed, simple and refined carbohydrates are quickly converted into energy. But that source of energy goes as fast as it comes. This leaves us feeling the need for a new source of energy, causing us to fix that with another source of quick acting energy, (refined or simple carbohydrates) and the circle goes on and on. This results in our bodies feeling the need to eat at all hours of the day.

This in turn, can lead us into other, more serious problems, since prolonged exposure to these types of carbohydrates cause the body to need to generate more insulin, resulting in our bodies becoming insulin-resistant. This means our bodies continue to need more and more insulin to compensate for our high blood sugar levels.

As you read about in the chapter on sugar, the first consequence of needing more insulin on a regular basis is that we begin to notice other functions of this hormone that are negatively impacted, such as the signal from our body to our brain letting it know that we are full and don't need to eat more. Due to the excess insulin this signal doesn't reach our brain and even though we don't need to, we keep eating more carbohydrates until we are on the verge of exploding.

Avoid industrial breads

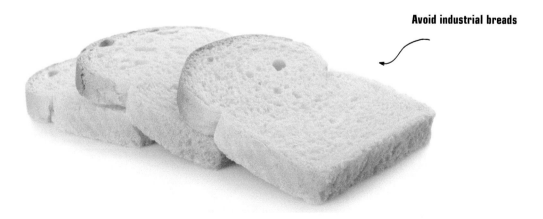

Has this ever happened to you?

The second consequence that we also saw in the chapter on sugar, is that if we end up becoming insulin-resistant then we are surely doomed to face one of these two scenarios below:

- Our blood sugar is totally **out of control** because our body is unable to generate the large amount of insulin it needs to control it, which most likely results in us having type 2 diabetes.

- Or, with our body **forcing itself** to generate greater amounts of triglycerides in order to help create the excess insulin needed, we become a higher risk for long-term cardiovascular disease.

Either of these two scenarios is very worrying.

In short, eating refined and simple carbohydrates might be the reason we are feeling the need to munch all the time. We eat more than we need and put ourselves at greater risk of getting sick in the long run. [Fig. 2].

WHO WINS AND WHO LOSES?

As is always the case, this change in our diet had a clear winner and a clear loser. So you tell me, if we remove a product that gives us a large amount of energy in small portions and is barely processed by the industry and we replace that product with another that causes us to lose control and eat more than we need plus it's cheap for the industry to process... who wins and who loses?

The winner is once again, the food industry. They found the perfect ingredient – refined carbs. With them, they can produce all kinds of cheap products that give them high margins of return. It's also a product that encourages the consumer to eat more than they need – sweet deal, right? It's such a successful business that the food industry has gone to great lengths to make sure that things stay like this for as long as possible. They have continually convinced western society that we should base our diet on a food pyramid where carbohydrates represent 60% of our total calorie intake. But we'll get into that in the next chapter.

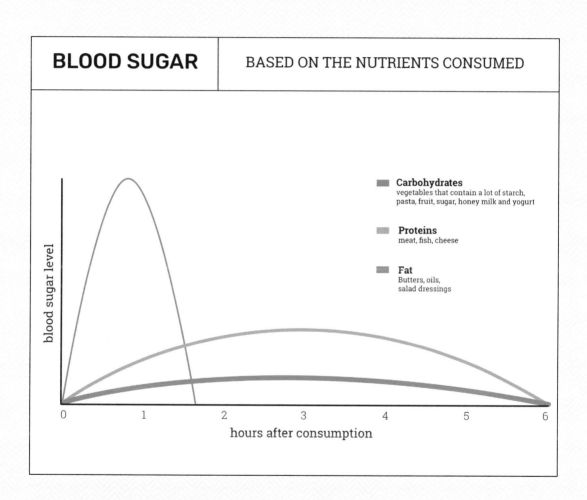

Figure 2: Carbohydrates are quickly converted into energy. However, their effects don't last long which causes us to need to find a new source of energy.

By following their system, we as consumers lose. However, all is not lost. Change is easy. We just have to stop listening to what the food industry says and start to listen to our own bodies.

To start with, we should pay attention to where our carbohydrates are coming from, that is, if we want to keep eating them of course. We should look for ones that have a 'slow release' composition so that instead of giving us this boost of energy, we get a steady supply of energy that is released little by little. This will help us to not feel hungry throughout the day and respect our bodies by not consuming more than we really need. Also, nutritionally speaking, these kinds of carbohydrates won't harm us and they will provide us with something more than just simple calories.

In other words, lets reduce as many of these 'fast acting carbs' and their derivatives as we can (white bread, flour, pasta, pastries etc.) – all of those things that have been modified so much so that not only do they provide us with no nutritional value, but in fact harm us. For example, a great alternative to cereals is to eat nuts. Change

Nuts are a great source of energy

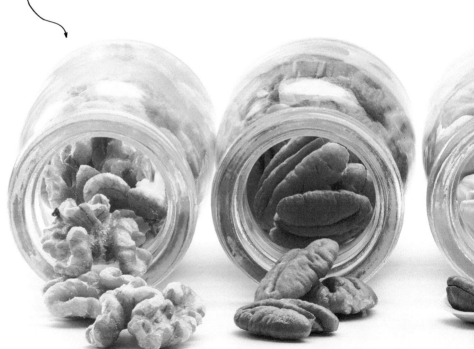

the conventional potato or rice that don't give you any nutrients and are just empty calories to something delicious like a sweet potato or quinoa – anything, that hasn't been modified over the years and still retains its nutrients. Eat fruit instead of drinking processed juices. That way you can really get all the fibre and other benefits they provide. And, most importantly let's increase the number of vegetables we eat. Many of them are nutrient-rich carbo-hydrates. They have infinite benefits to the human body, one of which is fibre. Basically, let's cut out all processed foods!

At first your body might crave them, and it may seem more difficult than it really is. It's normal.

Deep down, these carbs are sugars and they become addictive. However, if we stay consistent and turn towards fat as a natural source of energy then in two or three weeks, we will notice that we don't crave carbs like we once did and we will break that cycle of addiction. We will also begin to feel more energised, better rested and we will be in a better mood overall. What more could we want?

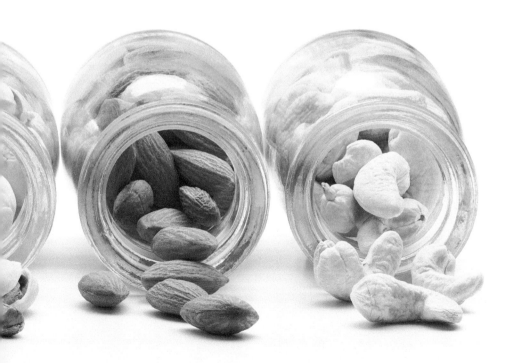

OTHER FOOD MYTHS

BESIDES THE PROBLEMS with carbohydrates, sugar and the deceptions about fats, there are three other myths related to the western food pyramid that also need to be addressed.

THE FIRST MYTH: USING THE FOOD PYRAMID AS THE BASIS OF A HEALTHY AND ADEQUATE DIET

The food pyramid is a visual representation used by the authorities in each country to indicate the recommended amounts of each food group to obtain a healthy diet. So, at the base of the food pyramid are the foods that we are supposed to eat in larger quantities and at the top are the foods that we should eat the least of.

Although each country and each agency offers its own food pyramid, they have all been quite similar and greatly influenced by the one the United States Department of Agriculture (USDA) published in 1992. Let's take a brief look to see what their recommendations are and, what they are based on.

Up until 1956 there were various recommendations made to society which basically consisted of dividing food groups into four, six or seven categories and then suggesting to consume various amounts of each said category.

However, in 1977, thanks to the popularity of Ancel Keys and other scientists who promoted the benefits of a low-fat diet, and due to the pressure from the food industry, particularly the Sugar Association, the US government published the 'Dietary Goals for the United States', where it was recommended to minimise the consumption of fats and cholesterol and increase our intake of carbohydrates, making them 55-60% of our total caloric intake (Select Committee on Nutrition and Human Needs 1977).

In 1992 the USDA designed its first food pyramid, which visually reflected the recommendations the government had been making since 1977. In the original version of the American food pyramid, the base food group was fruits and vegetables, not cereals and other derivatives. Of course, as we now know this was quickly modified due to the pressure from the entire food industry. This is the official food pyramid published in 1992.

USDA Pyramid, (1992)

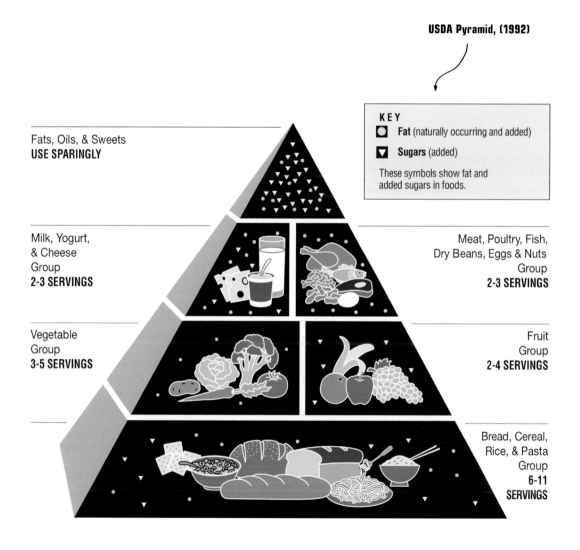

KEY

⬜ **Fat** (naturally occurring and added)

🔻 **Sugars** (added)

These symbols show fat and added sugars in foods.

Fats, Oils, & Sweets
USE SPARINGLY

Milk, Yogurt, & Cheese Group
2-3 SERVINGS

Meat, Poultry, Fish, Dry Beans, Eggs & Nuts Group
2-3 SERVINGS

Vegetable Group
3-5 SERVINGS

Fruit Group
2-4 SERVINGS

Bread, Cereal, Rice, & Pasta Group
6-11 SERVINGS

The final layout of the 1992 American food pyramid looked like this:

- The base (45-55% of daily consumed calories) was made up of breads, cereals, pastas, and rice.

- The next tier were vegetables (10-20%) and fruit (7-15%).

- The tier after that were dairy products (7-10%) and then meats, poultry, fish, eggs, legumes and nuts (another 7-10%).

- And finally, at the top were the fats and added sugars, although in this case they did not provide any recommended amounts.

Although the first food pyramid was published in a Swedish magazine back in 1974, it was the American one that popularised the concept around the world, and it was quickly adopted by most other countries.

In Spain, the first published version was in 2004 by the Spanish Society of Community Nutrition, although they presented some differences with that of the American 1992 version. For example, they separated the consumption of meat from fish, poultry, eggs, legumes and nuts. But nonetheless, everything was still practically the same.

As we can see, this standardised nutrition model that has been around since the 80s prioritised the consumption of cereals and other derivatives as the basis of our diet, again, making up 60% of our total diet.

It is still surprising to me to see how far the interests of the industry prevail over our own. It never ceases to amaze me to see that rice, cereals, and other such things as bread and pasta take up the most important place on the food pyramid. It is mind boggling.

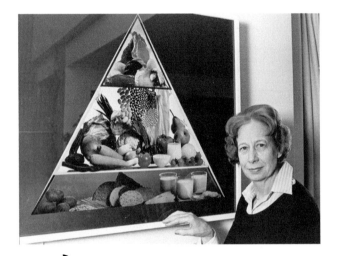

**Swedish Food Pyramid
1974**

Even more so when you stop to think that humans have eaten vegetables, proteins, nuts, fruits and berries throughout 99% of our history here on Earth.

And, as if that is not enough, we have a large number of published studies that show a diet high in fruits, and vegetables helps to protect us against diseases and improves our overall nutrition. One of the latest studies from Imperial College London, shows that we can even further protect ourselves against diseases by increasing the number of fruits and vegetables we eat to eight pieces a day.

Pyramid of the Spanish Nutrition Community Society (2004)

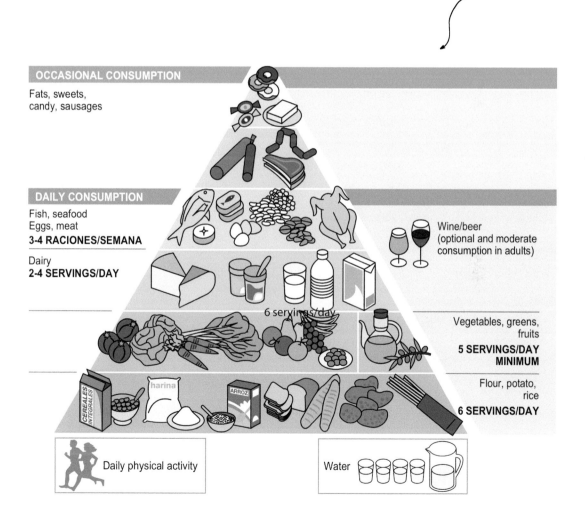

OCCASIONAL CONSUMPTION

Fats, sweets,
candy, sausages

DAILY CONSUMPTION

Fish, seafood
Eggs, meat
3-4 RACIONES/SEMANA

Dairy
2-4 SERVINGS/DAY

Wine/beer
(optional and moderate
consumption in adults)

6 servings/day

Vegetables, greens,
fruits
**5 SERVINGS/DAY
MINIMUM**

Flour, potato,
rice
6 SERVINGS/DAY

Daily physical activity

Water

It blows my mind when I look at the top of the food pyramid. How is it possible that sweets, pastries and even candy have a place on this pyramid but, fundamental nutrients such as fats which are necessary for our well-being, health and development are hardly represented? Of course, at this point we shouldn't be surprised at the lengths to which the food industry will go to promote their product or the collusion that goes on between them and the authorities, but needless to say, it infuriates me.

A food pyramid where profits are more important than the well-being of human life.

A food pyramid that prioritised the health and well-being of a person would disregard the economic profitability for the industry and would instead promote the intake of more fruits, vegetables and nuts. Followed by meat, poultry, fish, shellfish, eggs and fats.

These are the fundamental dietary changes that I suggest in my new project, Natruly. A diet that helps us to listen to our body which in turn, helps us to bring out the best of ourselves and continue to evolve. A diet like the one human's have been eating for the last 2.8 million years. [Fig. 3].

SECOND MYTH. IT'S BEST TO EAT 5 TIMES A DAY

For many years now we have been led to believe that the key to losing weight is to eat every 3 to 4 hours in order to keep our metabolism active and to help us avoid feeling overly hungry at mealtime, which would lead us to overindulging without much control.

The reality, however, is that this is a myth. It is an idea that has been based on the current high carb/low-fat, low-fibre model. A model which creates the need to constantly eat and keeps us from properly stimulating the hormone that helps us feel full.

The key to a healthy diet is to provide our body with the adequate nutrients it needs and to provide us with enough energy until our next meal, whenever that may be.

Consuming larger amounts of fat provides us with a greater feeling of satiety and longer-lasting energy – although, we still need to incorporate vitamins, minerals, antioxidants and fibre into our diet as well as proteins and some carbohydrates (unrefined, of course).

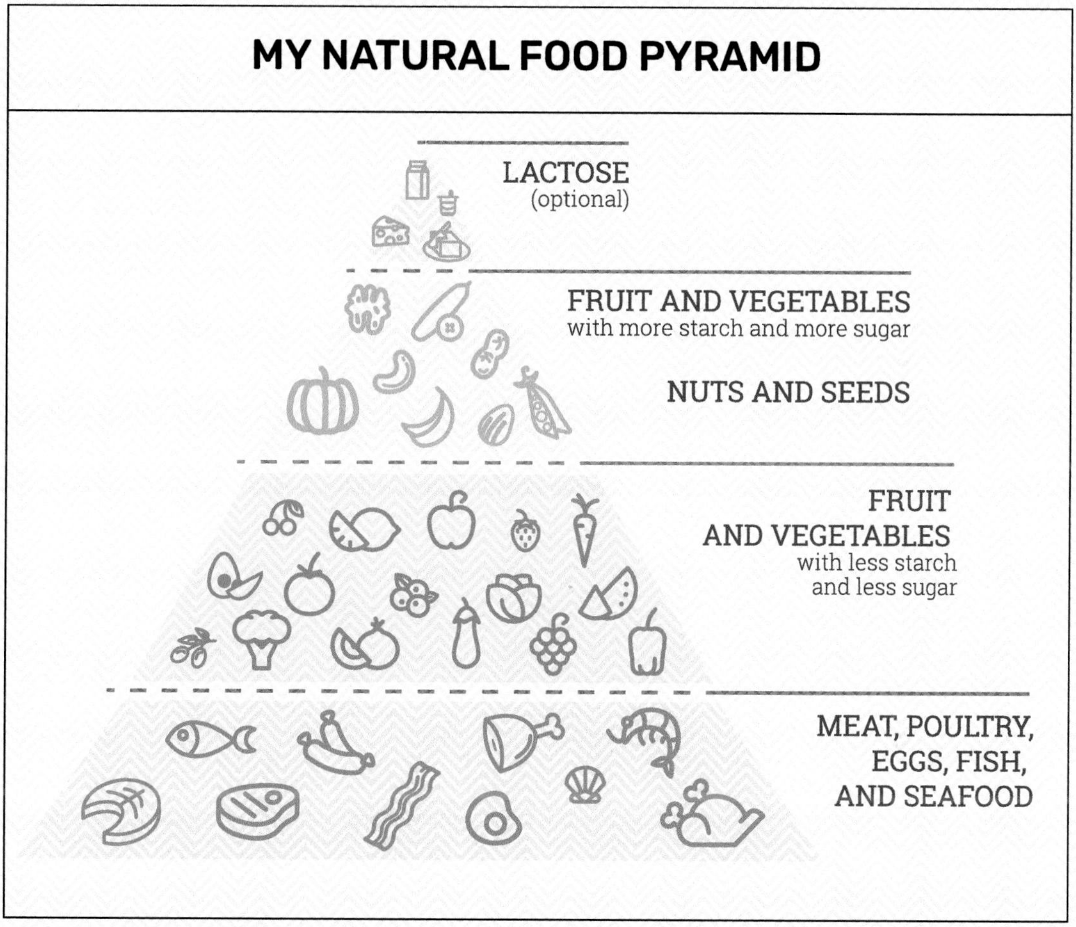

MY NATURAL FOOD PYRAMID

LACTOSE
(optional)

FRUIT AND VEGETABLES
with more starch and more sugar

NUTS AND SEEDS

FRUIT
AND VEGETABLES
with less starch
and less sugar

MEAT, POULTRY,
EGGS, FISH,
AND SEAFOOD

Figure 3: At Natruly, we have put together a food pyramid that is designed to promote health and well-being. Our pyramid is founded on: fruits, vegetables, nuts, berries, proteins and fats.

When it comes to your diet, the important thing is not the number of times you eat but rather the quality of the meals you are eating. Our body doesn't need to be 'activated' through eating food every few hours, rather it needs enough fuel to function properly. I mean think about, do you think humans a million years ago were able to eat 5 times a day?

Also, skipping a meal like breakfast every now and again is good. If we are constantly eating, our digestive system never gets a chance to rest. Leading us to our third myth.

THIRD MYTH. BREAKFAST IS THE MOST IMPORTANT MEAL OF THE DAY.

Even though more and more nutritionists argue that there is no reason for breakfast to be considered the most important meal of the day, there are still legions of people who continue to insist that not eating a large enough breakfast or worse, skipping breakfast is bad for your health and will leave you depleted of energy.

These breakfast advocates continue to advise people using a very interesting 'formula': juice + coffee with skimmed milk or chocolate with skimmed milk (for children but also many adults) + toast, breakfast cereal or cookies.

That is to say, a breakfast that only provides you with a lot of sugar, very little fibre, no fat, few vitamins and again more sugar. Juice, industrial chocolate-milk powder, cereal, cookies and toast are all foods that cause a large spike in insulin, which keeps us from feeling full and makes us eat more than we actually need. It just gives us an excessive amount of sugar, with hardly any nutrients. It is a cheap, harmful and short-lived source of energy that the body quickly absorbs and which activates the brain's pleasure zone.

It has not really been proven that you need to have a large breakfast when you wake up or that skipping breakfast prevents you from starting the day feeling energised or that it will cause you to have a nutritional deficit. Much less so, if you follow the breakfast menu like the one described above. This is once again a rule that has been thrust upon us by the food industry.

It would be more than enough if you had a little protein, fibre and/or fat to start the day. But it is neither mandatory nor will it make you healthier. What would be a great way to start your day is to ensure that you are well rested and that you have got your body accustomed to consuming foods that provide you with nutrients, thus ensuring that your body is functioning at 100%.

In other words, having a big breakfast isn't mandatory if you give your body what it needs throughout the rest of the day.

However, if you are someone who likes to start the day with something to eat like a piece of fruit with some toasted hazelnuts, or a couple of scrambled eggs cooked in butter with a little avocado on the side, then you will like my recipe section dedicated to healthy breakfast ideas.

It hasn't been proven that a large breakfast is necessary, the important thing is to be well rested and to get your body accustomed to consuming appropriate foods.

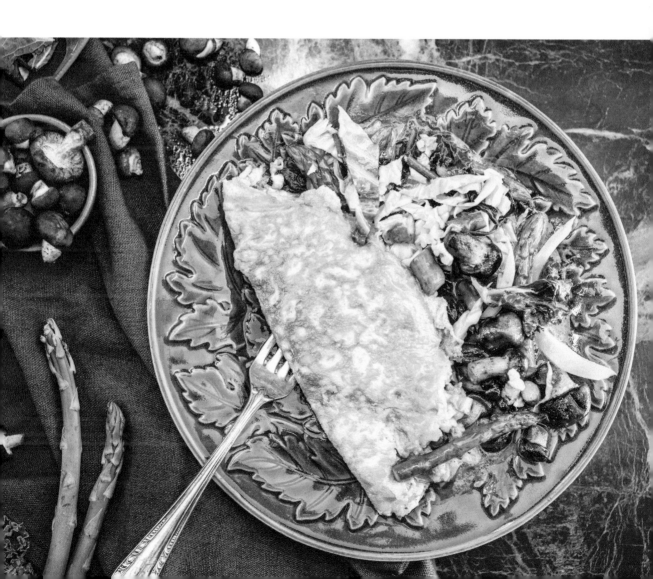

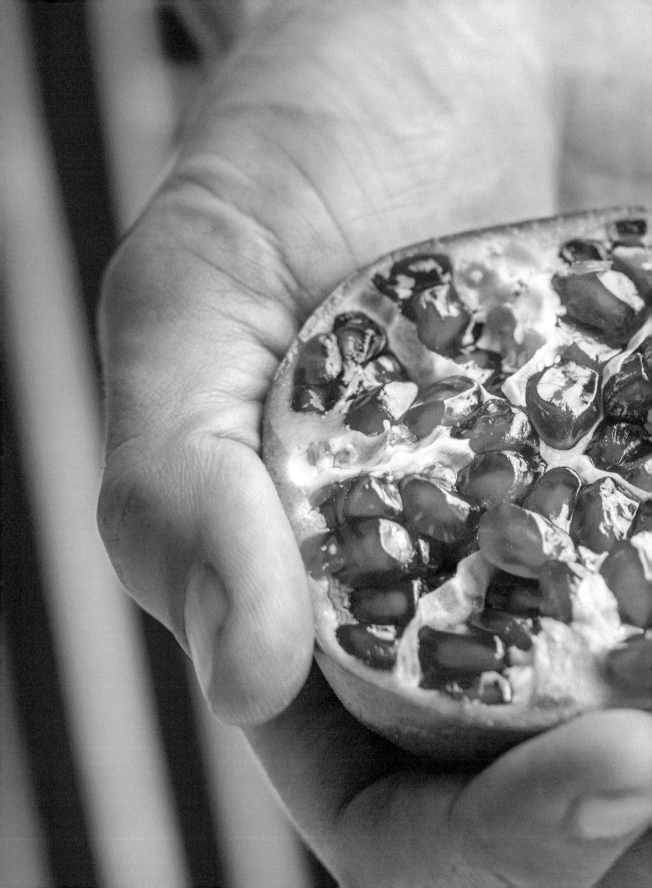

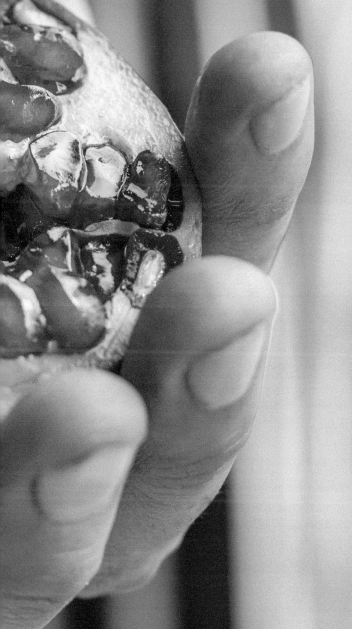

BEYOND THE
PALEO DIET

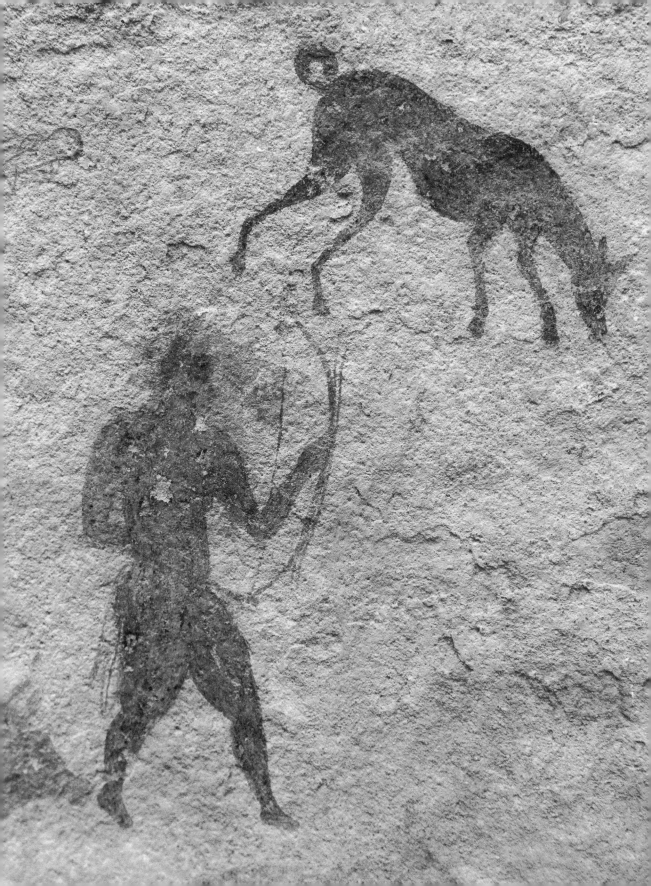

NOT SO LONG AGO, Americans came up with this trend of imitating what our ancestors did to take care of their body, as dictated by our 'core', it is known as the Paleo lifestyle.

For almost 3 million years, human beings maintained a diet that evolved over time along with their genes. A diet and a lifestyle that made us evolve and develop unlike any other species. It was a diet based on proteins, vegetables, fruit, fats and fibre. A diet which we started to modify 10,000 years ago and one which the food industry began distorting 50 years ago.

The Paleo diet is based on imitating the diet of our ancestors. Returning to our origins and looking to the past in order to help us get back on the right track.

And, while the Paleo diet is a great base to start with, we must go further.

Much further. It is not simply about foods we can and cannot eat. We don't have to exactly imitate what our ancestors did and ate 15,000 years ago. What's more, the vegetables and fruits of today have little to do with those that existed 15,000 years ago. We have redesigned and modified all of them. We couldn't go back even if we wanted to.

For almost three million years human beings had a diet based on proteins, vegetables, fruits, fats, and fibre.

What we really have to do is to get back on the right track. We need to eat as though our diet had evolved in the correct way and as if we had never fallen off the wagon. We need to go back to listening to our body and be aware of what feels good to us and what doesn't. This is different for everyone. By doing this, we will see that, in essence and broadly speaking, we find similar results. It is time to say NO to ultra-processed food, no to refined carbs and no to refined sugars. And say YES to vegetables, protein, fruits, nuts and natural fats.

We must focus, not only on our diet but also on rest and being in contact with nature. We need to learn how to appreciate the outdoors again; to enjoy each other and the world around us. In short, change our lifestyle. By doing so we will have learned to listen to our body and know what it needs on all levels. Therefore, we will be able to give it that without damaging or harming it.

We will start to notice that we have more and more energy, that we are getting less and less sick and that we feel better and are generally more animated and cheerful on a daily basis. In a nutshell, we'll be happier.

Who could really be opposed to this?

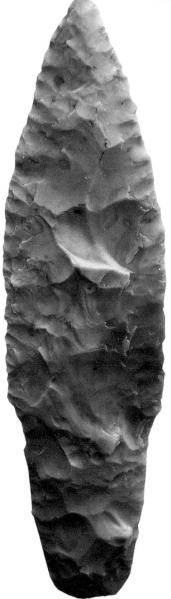

It has been a long time since we were hunter-gatherers and we have done many things incorrectly.

OUR ORIGINS

THE PALEOLITHIC ERA BEGAN 2.8 million years ago and ended about 10,000 years ago. Just 300 generations. It is at the end of the Paleolithic era that humans are considered to have gone from hunter-gatherers to pastoralism, where we developed agriculture, maintained livestock and became sedentary.

This change was of vital importance. First of all, there was a population explosion, but perhaps it was not done 'correctly'. We stopped feeding ourselves with what nature provided and started doing what was more comfortable for us.

We grew the crops that gave us the highest yield and ate the animals that we were able to domesticate. We made sure we had food, but was it the right kind of food?

During the almost 3 million years of the Stone Age, the physiology, metabolism and genetics of humans underwent massive transformations and evolved tremendously until we reached what we are today: Homo sapiens. Little has changed since then. Although the world has undergone many transformations over the last 10,000 years, thanks to the development of civilisation and its advances, genetically we have hardly evolved.

On the other hand, our diet has changed immensely over the last 10,000 years and the change – particularly over the last 50 years – has been quite radical and extremely worrying. We have gone from a diet and way of life that made us evolve and helped us to develop as a species, to a nutritionally poor diet and sedentary lifestyle. A diet and way of life that makes us sick instead of healthy.

The diet of the Paleolithic era depended on where groups lived and what time of year it was. The diet was based on the natural annual seasons and geographical location. It was a diet based on the natural maturation cycle of a given plant and animals that freely lived in the wild and who themselves ate a natural diet. It was a nomadic, hunter-gatherer lifestyle that forced us to move around. A truly natural lifestyle and diet.

After that, we started to eat the same foods all year long. We cultivated foods that were convenient to grow but not necessarily rich in nutrition. We began to eat fruits and vegetables that were grown in over-exploited plantations and farms and we started to consume artificially fattened animals. All of this was coupled with the fact that we stopped moving around. We started to reduce our physical activity so much so that today we hardly move at all.

The consequences of all those drastic changes in our diet and in our way of living was so severe that at the beginning of the Neolithic era, life expectancy went from 33 years old to 20 years old. That is a decrease of almost 50%.

Life expectancy can also be misleading since, if we disregard infant mortality and violent deaths, the life expectancy during the Paleolithic era could have been up to 70 years old, because at the time there were hardly any known diseases. This is in contrast to later on, with the development of agriculture, cattle ranching and a sedentary life where we have seen higher rates of diseases, epidemics and famines all of which have damaged our progression and genetic evolution.

Farming and the development of agriculture changed our lifestyle and our diet.

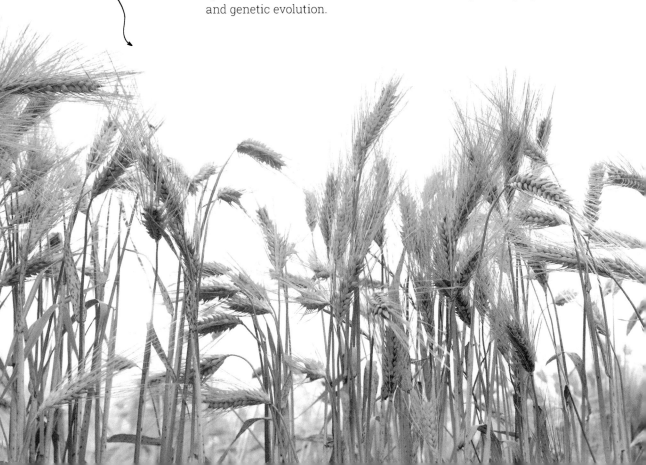

Life expectancy through the ages:

Period	Life Expectancy
Upper Paleolithic	33
Neolithic	20
Bronze Ages	18
Ancient Greece	20–30
Ancient Rome	20–30
Middle Ages	20–30
Early 20th Century	30–40
Early 21st Century	70

Fuente: Kaplan H. (2000): A Theory of Human Life, pp. 156-185.

Not only did life expectancy get worse but there were declines in other areas as well. The average height of someone during the Paleolithic era was over 1.77 metres for men and 1.66 for women – a height that is not common, even today. Also, our bone composition, teeth and even our brains were weakened by the change in diet and of lifestyle.

Think of how far we would be able to go if we were able to get back to the natural eating habits of our ancestors.

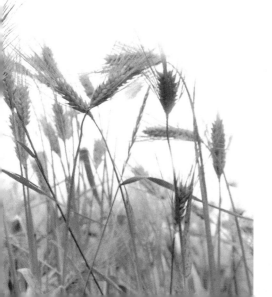

THE NATURAL EVOLUTION OF
THE PALEOLITHIC DIET

WE ALREADY KNOW THAT 10,000 years ago we began to change our way of life which led us to where we are today. We have made many mistakes along the way. If the history of humanity was represented by someone who is 85 years old, then the last 10,000 years would be like 3 months of that person's life. Which is to say, in the last 3 months we have adopted a harmful diet and lifestyle which isn't suited to us and makes us sick. [Fig. 4].

HOMO SAPIENS OF TODAY

Changing our habits, our way of life and our diet may seem more complicated than it really is. This is because the society in which we live seems to like to make things difficult for us; but we must take action. The consequences if we don't will be dire.

Diseases associated with a sedentary lifestyle and a poor diet have drastically increased in the last 50 years to an alarming rate. Although this process and its consequences began at the same time as the agricultural revolution it worsened and became more apparent during the industrial revolution 200 years ago. Since changing our nomadic lifestyle and diet during the Paleolithic era we have adopted what we now know as the 'Western Diet' which consists of a less nutritional diet and less physical activity.

The figures speak for themselves; the leading cause of death in Spain, where I live, is cardiovascular disease, followed by cancer and respiratory diseases. People who are overweight account for 50% of the adult population and 40% of children, which is very frightening (OECD 2020).

The interesting thing about all this is that with greater access to food and nutritional resources, the more dietary information we have at our disposal, the more professionals we have who specialise in guiding our eating habits and helping us to create a

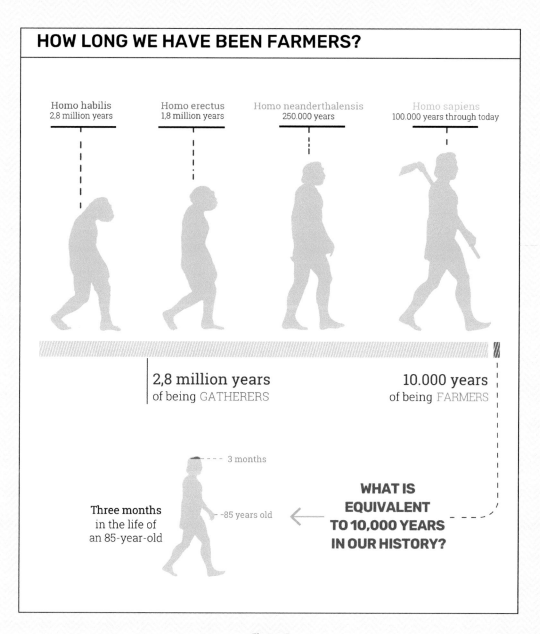

HOW LONG WE HAVE BEEN FARMERS?

Homo habilis
2,8 million years

Homo erectus
1,8 million years

Homo neanderthalensis
250.000 years

Homo sapiens
100.000 years through today

2,8 million years
of being GATHERERS

10.000 years
of being FARMERS

3 months

85 years old

Three months
in the life of
an 85-year-old

WHAT IS
EQUIVALENT
TO 10,000 YEARS
IN OUR HISTORY?

Figure 4

better lifestyle, illnesses relating to food keeping getting worse. So, what is the problem? Where did we go wrong?

There are many factors that have contributed to this problem, but the main factor is that we have put economic interests before the health interests of people. The lack of continuity between health professionals plays into the local interests of each player in the food industry, which results in countless nutritional guidelines by various international entities who differ in opinion.

Health-related associations support the consumption of ultra-processed foods that are known to be harmful to people because of the economic benefits they receive. To take Spain, where I live, these include endorsements to the Spanish Society of Cardiology from AvenaCol cookies; the endorsement to the Spanish Society of Diet and Science from Bollycao or the endorsement to the Spanish Pediatric Society from Dinosaurus cookies and/or Chocapic.

It is easy to guess who profits from people's poor health and poor eating habits.

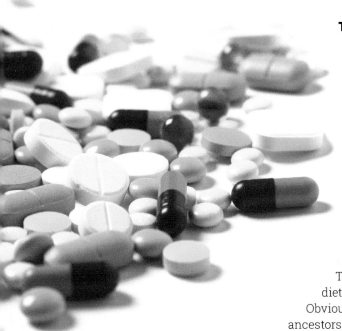

Furthermore, an unhealthy society also needs more drugs, and that doesn't hurt the pharmaceutical industry either. Even so, the main beneficiary of all this, without a shadow of a doubt, is the food industry, a global powerhouse. The more we eat, the worse we get, but they — they make more money.

Does that seem fair to you?

THE NATURAL EVOLUTION

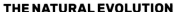

Despite all this, there is still hope. The last 10,000 years is just a drop in the ocean when it comes to the evolution of humans, which means there is still time to reverse our current predicament.

We are our cells. Our genetic material is what defines us and it is waiting for us to get back on track and return to the correct way of living so we can move forward in our development.

The reality is that we can't just change our diet — our lifestyle must change as well. Obviously, we can't eat and live exactly how are ancestors did, and I don't think we should. Regardless of what has happened, we are here now and, it is right

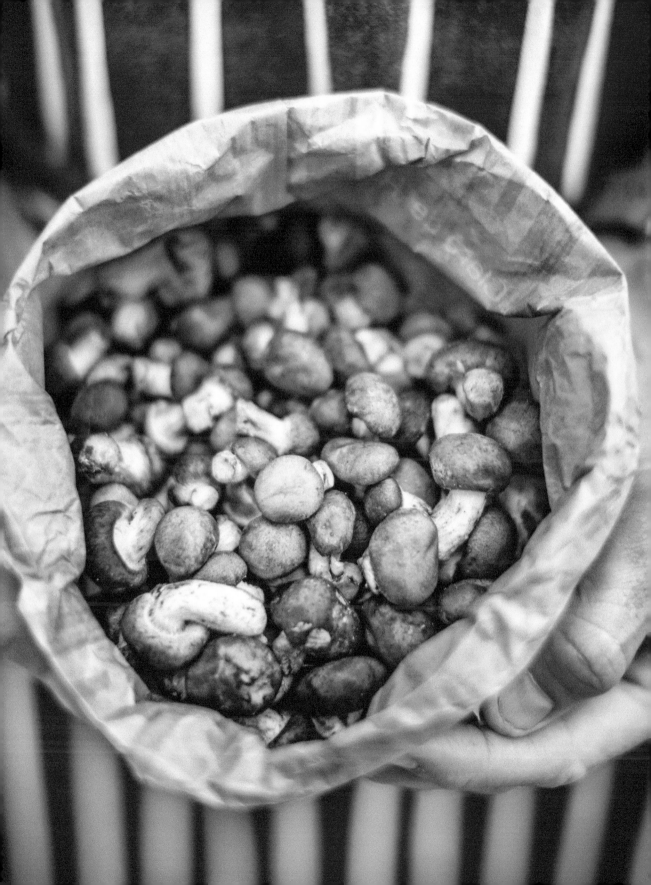

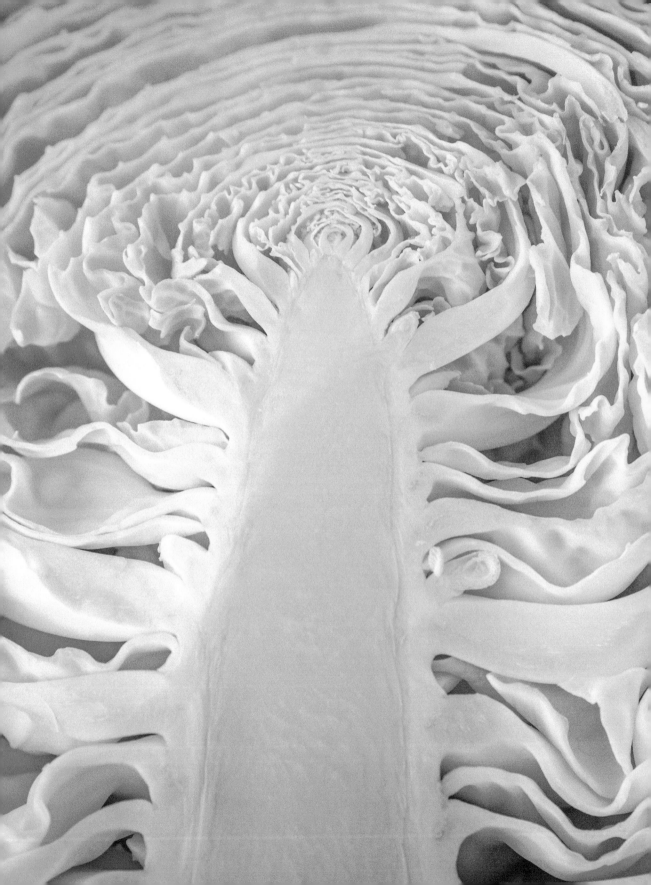

now in this moment that we can choose how we live and how we nourish ourselves.

So, do we try and lead a more active life? Or, do we allow ourselves to be sucked in by an industry and society that gives us short-term comfort for the here and now, with no regard for our health? Do we consciously make an effort to nourish ourselves thinking about our future well-being? Or, do we conform to the unhealthy current societal norms? Do we take actions to lead to a better life, or do we succumb to whatever society and the industry imposes on us?

Natural evolution is easy. It is about taking advantage of the knowledge we have gained and about getting back to our roots and eating those foods that made us strong and healthy.

Natural evolution is still a goal within our reach: you have to get back to eating the foods that made us healthy and strong.

We have to get back to eating the foods that promoted the proper functioning of our body. Go back to what feels good to us. The recipe for this is simple. Eat natural foods, listen to your body, cut out ultra-processed food, ignore the out-of-date and incorrect food pyramid and pay attention to what your body tells you. Forget about following a diet to lose weight. Forget about counting calories and let's start evaluating our food for its nutritional qualities and for what it gives our body.

Luckily, we have the tools to do just this. Listen to your body, pay attention to the signals it sends you, either in the form of pain, discomfort, lack of appetite or whatever it may be and get back on the right track. Let's get back to our roots and take advantage of the lessons we've learned.

THE BENEFITS OF A NATURAL DIET

Eating a natural diet isn't just a way of cooking, or a way to consume your food, it is a lifestyle change. It is about trying to get back to the ways of our ancestors. Giving our body what feels good, based on a diet that we were genetically designed for, with the aim of improving on our current quality of life. It is a diet based on eating fruits and vegetables, healthy fats, quality protein and having a respect for nature. Let's take a look at what the benefits are when you make this lifestyle change.

IMPROVE YOUR FITNESS LEVEL: MORE MUSCLE, LESS FAT

It has been shown through various studies that following a natural diet, that eliminates ultra-processed foods, sugars, and refined carbs improves a person's body composition, regardless of whether the person is already overweight or if they are at an appropriate weight for their age and sex.

Body fat decreases as a result of following a natural diet. This is thanks to the increased consumption of healthy fats and the elimination of refined carbohydrates and sugars. This is how we get our body to stop using carbohydrates as its main source of fuel and to start using fat in their place, the most abundant source of energy reserves we have in our body.

Being more physically active is also important in living a natural lifestyle along with consuming quality proteins. That way you don't lose your muscle mass, and in fact it might even increase despite losing weight. When I started living this lifestyle, I lost 4 kilos (about 8.8 pounds or 0.62 stone). I am 191 cm tall/ 6 feet 2 inches.

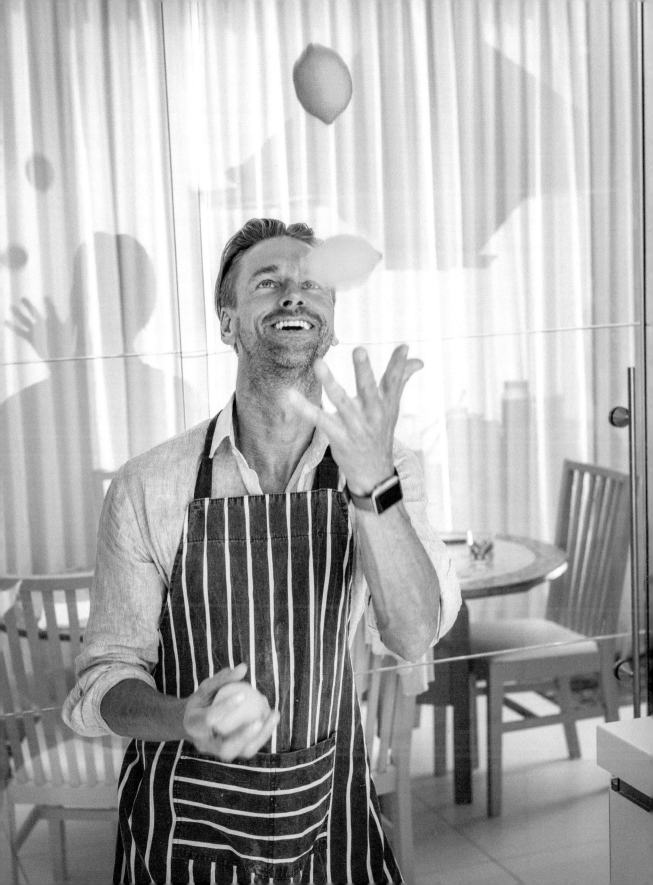

SLEEP BETTER

Quality sleep is another aspect that we have to improve nowadays. The pace of life today is so fast and it doesn't give us the opportunity to take naps, which is why a good night's sleep is essential to health. Taking a nap is wonderful and very healthy for those lucky enough to do it. However, if you are one of those who are unable to do so, don't worry because eating a natural diet will also help you to improve the quality of your sleep and guarantee that you get a good night's rest.

Cutting out sugars and refined carbs has been closely linked to better quality sleep.

Cutting out sugars and refined carbohydrates from your diet is directly related to improved, quality sleep. Let's dive a little deeper and see why. The hormone that is responsible for making us fall asleep is called melatonin.

Humans produce it naturally, but it depends on your tryptophan, which is an amino acid widely found in a Paleo diet (it is present in eggs, seeds, meat and, to a lesser extent, dried fruit.) Thus, by favouring the correct synthesis of melatonin, improved sleep follows. In addition to producing more melatonin, by making smaller portioned, satiating meals you won't find yourself going to bed with a bloated belly or the feeling of being stuffed.

BOOST YOUR DIGESTIVE SYSTEM

The majority of people associate fibre with cereal. However, they aren't the only foods that provide us with fibre. Vegetables, fruits and seeds that are prominent in the natural diet that I'm suggesting are all full of fibre. We must take advantage of the fibre found in these foods and not of those in cereal.

Fibre plays an important role since it is the nutrient in charge of feeding our gut bacteria, which promotes the growth of healthy bacteria that fight against other pathogens. Combining a sugar-free diet with a diet rich in fibre and free from refined carbohydrates guarantees a health microbiota (better known as gut flora). Of course, logically, this all has a direct impact on the overall state of our health.

Our intestinal flora is made up of bacteria; our digestive system contains about a kilo's worth. On the one hand they use the fibre to improve intestinal transit which promotes better and more frequent bowel movements, while on the other hand feeding itself by fermenting what we eat.

We also know that the derived chemical elements from the fermentation of fibre, proteins and fats help to maintain a healthy immune system. It is so important in fact that the intestinal microbiota has come to be known as the second human brain. Just another reason why it is important to take care of the ecosystem that inhabits our digestive system as its impact on our immune system and intestinal transit is vital.

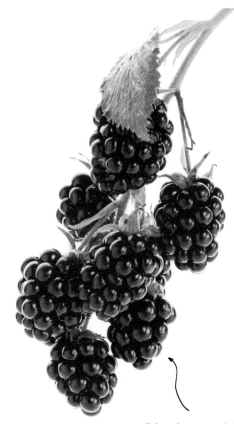

Take advantage of the fibre found in vegetables, fruits and seeds.

FEEL FULL LONGER: FIBRE, FAT AND PROTEIN

A natural diet based on vegetables, fruits, fats and proteins makes up a very satisfying and filling diet thanks to the composition of all the different nutrients each contain. Vegetables provide a lot of fibre. Different fats not only give you the feeling of being full but they also add flavour to your dishes. The feeling of fullness that you get from proteins is well known, since they are the macronutrients used in most 'miracle diets' in order for those who try these fads to not starve while attempting them.

By combining all these nutrients, we get the perfect 'satiating' formula. If fat and fibre are both present in some way in every meal, you are guaranteed to feel full. Like we saw before, it is impossible to get the same sensation with a diet based on refined carbohydrates and sugary processed foods.

IMPROVE THE FUNCTION OF YOUR PANCREAS

Once again, thanks to the elimination of sugars and processed foods that contain high amounts of refined carbohydrates, your pancreas will regain its strength and be healthier than ever. Basically, you will be resetting your sensitivity to insulin and by doing so, you will improve your body's response to this hormone and be able to maintain normal blood glucose levels.

The reason why is mainly because when we base our diet on vegetables, fats and proteins, we are respecting the pancreas's natural and normal fluctuations of insulin secretion.

After eating these kinds of foods, insulin increases slowly and progressively, unlike if you eat a diet that is rich in carbohydrates, sugars, and refined flours with a high glycemic index.

Continual consumption of those foods alters the secretion of insulin in your body which can lead a person to become resistant to this hormone. Insulin resistance causes major disorders, such as hyperglycemia, which is when your body is unable to control excess blood glucose levels despite the secretion of insulin. This causes a person to constantly crave food, even when your body doesn't need it. And, as we already spoke about, the long-term consequences of insulin resistance are being overweight, and having type 2 diabetes.

IMPROVE THE QUALITY OF FOOD YOU EAT

Cutting out sugar, cereal and some root vegetables from your diet doesn't mean you are going to starve. Actually, it means quite the opposite. As we know, the main supply of fuel for your body from now on is going to come from healthy fats. The supply of energy that comes from vegetables and fruits with low glycemic indexes such as that from berries, is gradually released into the body which prevents us from feeling hungry only a short while after eating.

Again, this is the opposite of what happen when you consume high glycemic carbohydrates, as we have seen before.

WHICH ARE THE BEST NATURAL FOODS?

THE KEY TO LEADING a healthy life is your diet. Exercise is of course very important as well; but regardless of how many sports you play or how active you are, if you don't take care of your diet the rest makes little difference.

Every product we consume forms the pillars of our health. Therefore, it is very important to choose wisely. There is a vast variety of fresh and natural products available to everyone at any price point, so there are no excuses.

Following a healthy diet in no way means giving up delicious meals. Many people falsely believe that eating healthy is synonymous with eating just raw vegetables and bland dishes. Or worse, they think that they just have a long list of restricted foods and that they are limited. Things couldn't be further from the truth. There are countless spices and ingredients that can be used to make flavourful dishes for all different types of cuisine. The only downside to eating healthy is that you have to put in a little more effort when filling up your shopping cart or eating out at a restaurant. That is because there are many ultra-processed foods, full of sugar, starch and hydrogenated fats out there, that we have to be cautious of. They don't nourish our body and can become addicting for many.

Living a natural lifestyle is a combination of many factors. One of these is the importance of knowing where our food comes from and knowing how to read labels.

You don't have to give up flavourful foods.

We should always opt for organic and eco-friendly products whenever we can. Additionally, all products both plant and animal have a natural life cycle which should be respected. Luckily, there are some fruits and vegetables which occur naturally throughout the year like chard, lettuce or carrots.

However, oranges, tomatoes and peppers among many others are seasonal fruits and vegetables. So, it is important that we as consumers are aware of a food's natural life cycle. That way, we can try to cause the least possible impact on the environment. We live in a very consumerist society where we have become used to finding whatever we want or need at any time of year

As consumers it is important that we are aware of that natural life cycles of food.

That excessive type of consumerism has led to the manipulation and alteration of a product's natural maturation process. It in turn affects the composition, taste and quality of the food we eat.

In any case, there is no doubt that the secret to making positive changes is to be as creative as possible. Just because you are choosing to eat healthy doesn't mean you have to settle.

You can still eat delicious meals. Have you ever tried apple with almond spread? If not, try it! It is amazing! If you live with your partner or family it is easier when everyone is participating in living a healthy lifestyle. So, don't be afraid to get your family involved. Have them make suggestions and decisions when shopping or cooking.

So, which foods are best? Let's break it down into groups. Below, you will see each individual food group and I will provide you with information to help you understand more about each one and how they can either benefit or harm you. Keep in mind that food can be different for everyone, and everyone has their preferences and might not always agree. This is to say, what's good for some doesn't necessarily have to be good for others. Stay open, try things and listen to your body.

VEGETABLES AND GREENS

Since the beginning of time, humans have gathered seeds, fruits, vegetables and greens which were their main sources of food.

There are a great number of vegetables and vegetable varieties to choose from. Each one tastes different and contain different kinds of nutrients. Most vegetables can be eaten raw, or cooked. They can be used as the main ingredient or as a garnish or side dish. They are very beneficial and good to eat at any time of day.

Things are simple with vegetables, just follow one very easy rule: make your plate colorful and switch it up by using different coloured vegetables when preparing a meal. That way you can ensure that you are consuming a diverse amount of nutrients.

Broccoli has a ton of fibre but it is better to eat it during winter.

Each vegetable and greens family has different nutritional properties. It's good to know each one's characteristics so that you can choose wisely.

- Cruciferous: broccoli, cauliflower, Brussel sprouts, Chinese cabbage, collard greens, radish, turnip, arugula and, watercress are some of many members of this group of vegetables. They are full of water, which is great for hydration, and loaded with fibre and vitamin B which are both vital for the proper functioning of our digestive system.

- Allium: leeks, onions, chives and garlic are all part of this veggie group which have healing properties. They are a natural diuretic and help regulate blood sugar levels.

- Nightshades: include tomatoes, aubergine, and peppers (including chillies). The best thing about these vegetables is that they provide us with many essential vitamins such as vitamin A, B and C along with various other minerals such as potassium, calcium, phosphorus and magnesium. They are perfect for keeping your bones and brain healthy.

- Leafy greens: chard, spinach, chicory, celery, endives, fennel, green beans and lettuce are just a small part of this expansive family of vegetables. They provide us with not only with large amounts of water (between 85-95%) but they also provide us with carotenes and folic acid (essential for pregnant women) as well as vitamin B and other minerals such as iron, iodine, calcium and potassium.

- Fresh herbs: thyme, parsley, coriander, basil, oregano, mint, arugula, and lamb's lettuce. These small plants are often used to flavour and season dishes. What makes them really stand out though is their antioxidant and hypotensive, anti-inflammatory and digestive properties. They are literally nature's medicine.

- Mushrooms: There are too many to list here, but a few favourites are portobellos, shitake, and cremini mushrooms. They are a great source of plant proteins and water. They are the perfect way for vegetarians and vegans to get the proteins they need. Additionally, they strengthen our immune system and provide many group B vitamins.

- Tubers and roots: out of all the groups listed these have the highest concentration of carbohydrates but they have a low starch index. These include sweet potatoes, cassavas, beetroots and yams (also known as squash). They are a good source of vitamin K which is good for our bones and vascular system. They also supply us with riboflavin and pantothenic acid which is great for your skin and hair.

Yams supply us with large amounts of Vitamin K.

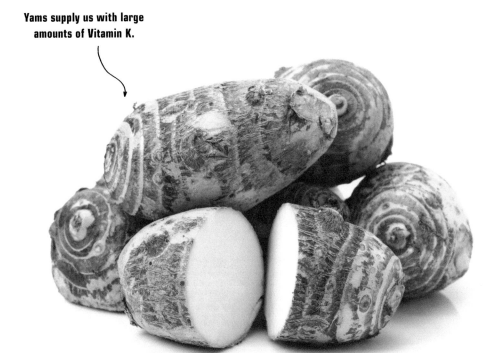

Vegetable	January	February	March	April	May	June	July	August	September	October	November	December
Artichoke						•	•	•	•			
Asparagus				•	•	•						
Aubergine							•	•	•			
Beetroot							•	•	•	•		
Broccoli	•	•	•	•	•	•	•	•	•		•	•
Brussels sprouts	•	•	•							•	•	•
Cabbage	•	•	•	•	•	•	•	•	•	•	•	•
Carrot	•	•	•	•	•	•	•	•	•	•	•	•
Cauliflower	•	•	•	•	•	•	•	•	•	•	•	•
Celery	•	•	•	•	•	•	•	•	•	•	•	•
Chard						•	•	•	•			
Courgette						•	•	•	•			
Cucumber	•	•	•	•	•	•				•	•	•
Endive	•	•						•	•	•	•	•
Escarole						•	•	•	•	•		
Green Beans						•	•	•				
Green Pepper			•	•	•	•	•	•				
Lamb's lettuce	•	•	•	•						•	•	•
Lettuce				•	•	•	•	•	•			
Leek	•	•	•	•							•	•
Mushroom									•	•		
Milk thistle	•	•				•	•	•				•
Onion								•	•			
Parsnip	•	•	•	•	•		•	•	•	•	•	•
Pumpkin									•	•	•	•
Red cabbage	•	•	•	•	•	•	•	•	•		•	•
Red pepper						•	•	•				
Spinach	•	•	•	•	•					•	•	•
Spring onion	•	•	•	•	•	•	•	•	•	•	•	•
Sprouts	•	•	•							•	•	•
Sweet potato	•	•	•							•	•	•
Tender garlic	•	•	•	•	•	•					•	•
Tomato	•	•	•	•	•	•	•	•	•	•	•	•
Turnip	•	•					•	•	•	•	•	•
Watercress					•	•	•	•	•	•	•	

Chart of seasonal vegetables

FRUITS

Our ancestors during the Paleolithic era collected the fruit that nature provided at any given season. They ate them for more than just their refreshing taste. Let's take a look at some of their benefits.

- They strengthen our immune system: thanks to the large presence of micronutrients they contain. This in turn helps to prevent diseases and to heal our body.

- Good for our skin: fruit contain large amounts of water which helps to keep our skin fresh, clean and, hydrated.

They are good and good for you, but it is important to remember to eat in season fruit and not to over-indulge because of their high fructose content.

Not all fruits are created equal, some provide us with more energy than others, some may contain more fibre than another etc. Citrus fruits for example are a great source of vitamin C and citric acid. The medical and cosmetic benefits of this kind of fruit have been well known and documents for centuries; but did you know it is also a good source of biofuel?

And, wild fruits, those tiny fruit that grow on bushes are mini antioxidant bombs thanks to their high content of vitamin C, anthocyanins and carotenoids. These last two nutrients are often the reason why wild fruits are called superfoods or nutrient bombs.

The best thing about fruit is obviously that they have wonderful nutritional properties. They are a great source of natural carbohydrates, fibre, vitamins, minerals and of course, water. Fruit makes it easy to get creative. You can add them to savoury dishes or use them in desserts for a natural sweet taste or we can whip up some delicious smoothies by mixing several kinds together. In just a single glass we can be both refreshed and nourished with all-natural nutrients!

Below I have provided a list of fruits organised according to their glycemic index, which is to say the amount of carbohydrates contained in each kind.

GI Category	Fruit	January	February	March	April	May	June	July	August	September	October	November	December
Low GI 1 - 35	Almond										•	•	
	Apple	•									•	•	•
	Apricot					•	•	•	•	•			
	Avocado	•	•	•	•	•	•	•	•	•	•	•	•
	Blueberry						•	•	•	•			
	Cherry						•	•	•	•			
	Coconut			•	•	•							
	Custard apple					•	•	•	•	•			
	Fig	•	•	•	•	•	•	•				•	•
	Grapefruit	•	•	•	•	•						•	•
	Lemon	•	•	•	•	•	•	•	•	•	•	•	•
	Lime			•	•	•	•	•	•	•			
	Nectarine						•	•	•	•			
	Orange	•	•	•	•							•	•
	Peach							•	•	•			
	Pear	•							•	•	•	•	•
	Plantain	•	•	•	•	•	•	•	•	•			
	Plum							•	•	•			
	Pomegranate								•	•			
	Quince										•	•	•
	Raspberry					•	•	•					
	Tangerine	•	•	•	•							•	•
	Strawberry					•	•	•	•				
Medium GI 36 - 50	Date								•	•			
	Grape								•				
	Kiwi								•	•			
	Mango					•	•	•					
	Persimmon										•	•	•
	Pineapple	•	•	•									•
High GI 51 - 75	Cantaloupe						•	•	•				
	Loquat	•	•	•									•
	Papaya					•	•	•	•	•			
	Raisin						•	•					
	Watermelon			•	•	•	•	•	•	•			

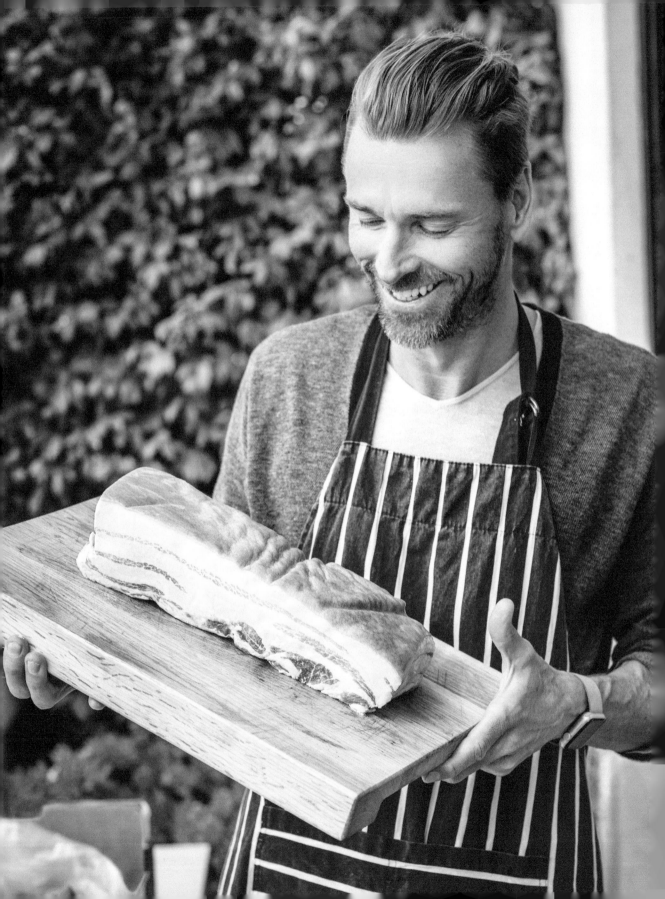

MEATS

The most common and easy-to-find meats are: poultry like chicken and turkey as well as beef like veal or ox. Pork is a remarkable ingredient particularly in Spanish gastronomy since they use every part of the pig. Some other popular lean meats are lamb and rabbit.

Another interesting and highly recommended source of protein comes from game meat. This has a very interesting nutritional composition. Some of the most well-known types of game are deer, goose, pheasant, quail, duck, pigeon, and wild boar. There are also other types of more exotic game but they can be harder to find. These are elk, turtle, kangaroo, emu, ostrich and bison. So, if you travel abroad you might want to keep an eye out for any of these.

Proteins from free-range, grass-fed animals are very beneficial to our health.

Iron and zinc are two nutrients that really stand out when eating beef, lamb, pork, and rabbit. Unfortunately, nowadays we don't use or eat every part of the animal like our ancestors did, which is a pity. For example, both liver and kidney either raw or cooked are very good and important sources of many vitamins and minerals.

Game meat and/or organs are great allies to eating a healthy diet because less adulterated hormones and antibiotics are used on them and they are richer in nutrients. Proteins that come from free-range, grass-fed animals are very beneficial to our health but, buying that kind of meat can sometimes be more difficult and more expensive.

Again, liver is an excellent alternative as it is a great source of protein and is much cheaper than other more expensive and less nutritious cuts of meat.

Let's breakdown the properties of meat:

- Water: between 60% and 80% of the weight of meat is water, which is key to staying hydrated.

- Proteins: are essential for healing our body and keeping it ready at all times. Proteins are responsible for forming and repairing muscle tissue, tendons, bones, skin, hair and all of our other organ tissues. Meat is comprised of between 20-25% protein of which 40% are essential amino acids that are body can only get through our diet.

- Fats: when people hear this word, they often want to run, but, as we have already seen, fats are good for our blood vessels and help to reduce the possibility of cardiovascular disease.

- Vitamins: meat is a great source of B vitamins, such as B1 (thiamine), B3 (niacin), as well as B6 and 12. Meat also provides us with vitamins A and E.

- Minerals: meats, depending on the kind you eat, are also wonderful sources of iron and zinc which is highly recommended for people who suffer from anaemia.

Meat has many beneficial properties. It can be eaten cooked or raw. The difference between eating it one way or the other is mainly due to the molecular structure of the protein as it changes when we manipulate it. It starts to dilute itself, breaking it down, which makes it easier to digest.

Meat can lose some of its essential nutrients depending on how we prepare it. This is mainly due to the meat sweating when cooked. You can help to prevent this by sealing the meat or cooking it at high temperatures. The water or juice that is released when the meat is cooked contains many of the nutrients and can be used as a broth or sauce.

Meat provides us with essential amino acids.

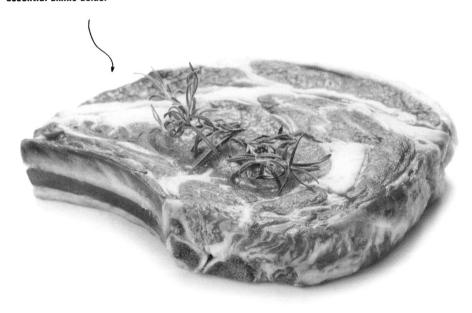

FISH AND SEAFOOD

Foods from the sea such as fish, shellfish and molluscs are loaded with minerals and essential fatty acids including omega-3s, calcium and phosphorus.

They also have other fantastic nutritional properties – primarily the essential amino acids and proteins they provide – but they also contain a high concentration of valuable vitamins and minerals.

Seafood and fish provide us with essential amino acids, protein, calcium, phosphorus, fatty acids like the very beneficial and well-known omega-3.

Their nutritional properties help us fight against disease. They promote the improved function of the digestive system by regulating glucose and uric acid in the blood as well as fat. Great for people who suffer from diabetes or who have unbalanced cholesterol levels.

There are so many varieties of fish and seafood including molluscs and crustaceans.

Mediterranean gastronomy, especially from coastal regions is famous for its use of fish and seafood in an array of dishes:

- White fish: is one of the best quality proteins, it is light and provides us with calcium, iron, iodine, copper and phosphorus. These minerals are essential for children to properly grow. White fish include hake, monkfish, cod, seabass, perch, and grouper among others.

- Blue fish: contains necessary fatty acids which contain omega-3s that are very beneficial to our circulatory system thanks to their anti-inflammatory and blood-thinning properties. Blue fish include eel, herring, mackerel, swordfish, salmon, and sardines to name just a few.

- Shellfish: is an excellent option if you are looking to have a variety of choices in your diet. Shellfish have many health properties but among those that stand out are vitamins A, B and E which are all great antioxidants that help to improve our skin as well as providing women with essential folic acid during

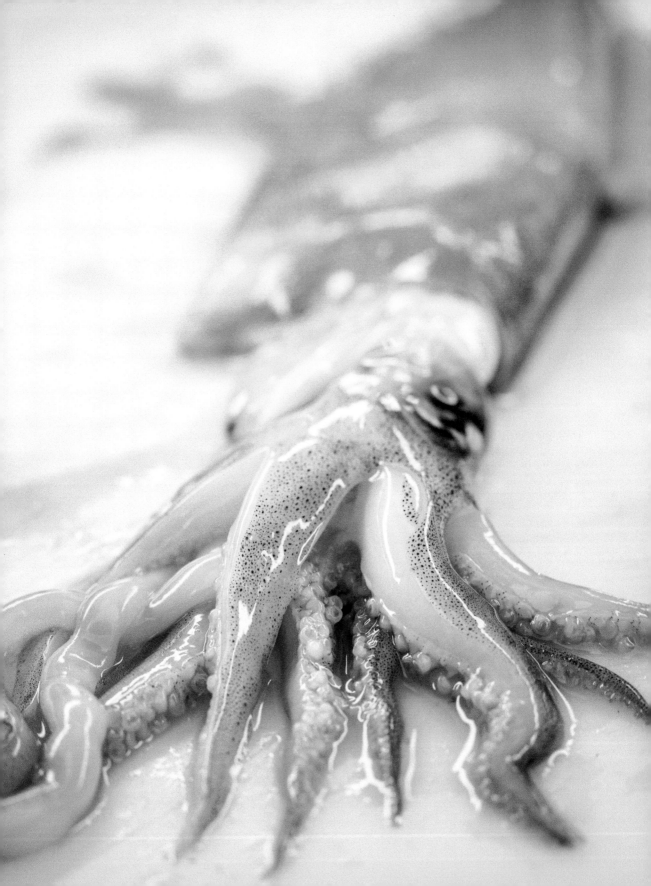

pregnancy, and also helps to prevent anemia. Shellfish contain a large presence of minerals such as potassium, iodine, magnesium and sodium. Clams, mussels and cockles also contain iron, and squid and prawns are a good source of calcium.

EGGS

Eggs are one of the most versatile foods in the kitchen. They provide us with seven different vitamins and more than five essential minerals, not to mention their wonderful composition of different fats. When it comes to choosing your eggs, it's best to opt for free-range or organic eggs. Make sure to look at the first number of the long code which can be found on the shell of the egg. Codes beginning with the numbers 1 or 0 come from free-range or organic chickens.

Eggs are widely used in cooking throughout the world. Although most of the eggs we consume come from chickens, eggs from other birds are also a great option.

Contrary to the popular belief that eggs increase our cholesterol level, they are actually very beneficial to our health:

- Nutrient rich: among them are proteins, health fats, minerals, and various antioxidants. They are also an especially good source of selenium, vitamin D, and riboflavin.

- Large presence of choline: Choline is an essential nutrient. This nutrient is required to make acetylcholine, an important neuro-transmitter which helps to keep our nervous system healthy. It also helps to transfer fat to tissues that need them and removes cholesterol from your liver. Consuming choline during pregnancy is especially important as it plays a similar role to folic acid.

Free-range egg codes start with the number 1 and organic eggs with the number 0. So, pay attention!

The recommended daily requirement for choline is 425 mg for women (when pregnant, 450 mg, and during lactation, 550 mg) and 550 mg for men in general. Can you guess how much choline is in one egg? The answer about 125mg – so you can see how important they are.

- Strengthens eyesight: eggs also contain lutein and zeaxanthin which are great antioxidants for your eyes because they rebuild the retina and reduce your chances of suffering from eye diseases such as cataracts.

- Good Source of vitamin D: vitamin D is directly related to the growth and development of our bones. However, it is famously difficult for our body to synthesise this vitamin and take advantage of its benefits. This is why vitamin D is known as the sunshine vitamin because exposure to its rays allows our body to absorb and synthesise this nutrient. In addition, vitamin D helps to regulate the body's use of minerals particularly calcium.

- Eggs don't negatively impact our blood cholesterol: the cholesterol we eat does not directly affect our blood cholesterol levels equally. Our liver produces large amounts of cholesterol every day. So, when we consume foods rich in cholesterol such as eggs, our liver then produces less of it which in turn creates a balance of the amount of cholesterol in our blood.

- May reduce heart disease: eggs have been demonised for many years as it was previously thought that they increase blood cholesterol levels and therefore contribute to heart-related diseases; however, this is not the case. Several studies have shown that there is no link between the consumption of eggs and heart disease or cardiac arrest.

NUTS AND SEEDS

Nuts and seeds are also highly nutritious foods that provide us with protein, fat, vitamins, and antioxidants. Adding them into our meals increases our dishes' nutritional value and gives us more variety in our diet. They both share similar characteristics – for example, they both contain less than 50% water, they are rich in fat, trace elements and protein which make them very energising. Some even contain vitamins and omega-3 fatty acids.

Nuts are amazing, tiny foods. They were very prominent and important in our ancestors' diet thanks to their energy and natural fat content. The best part was at that time they had not been altered or manipulated by humans. They are so good that you can even make flour with them. Needless to say, they are very beneficial to our health.

One of the best parts of nuts is that each one has a different flavour and nutritional contribution:

• Almonds: Traditional in Arabic dishes, almonds were popularised around the world a few hundred years ago. They contain omega-6s and are a good source of protein, carbohydrates and natural oils. They also provide us with vitamins B2 and E, magnesium, manganese and phosphorus. They help to reduce blood glucose levels which is great for those suffering from diabetes but also for those who aren't. They also contain antioxidants and help to make us feel full.

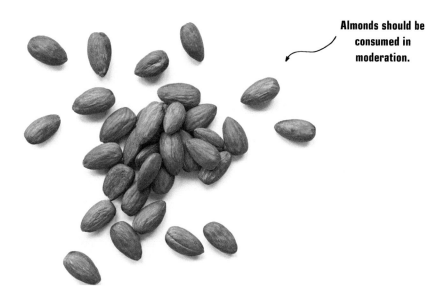

Almonds should be consumed in moderation.

The problem with almonds though is that there is a disproportionate balance between omega-6 and omega-3. However, if consumed in moderation, and combined with other foods like salmon, tuna or chia which contain omega-3s, then they aren't bad for you.

- Cashews: originally from Asia and Africa they are one of the fattiest and most hydrating nuts, although they don't provide much fibre. They contain vitamins K and E, iron, magnesium, manganese and phosphorus, beta-carotene and lutein.

It is important to note that cashews are the second most common nut responsible for causing allergies (only peanuts cause more, although technically they are a legume).

They also contain some of the highest amounts of carbohydrates compared to other nuts so again, they should be eaten in moderation.

- Hazelnuts: are not often eaten alone just like walnuts and pistachios as they are usually found in other products that we commonly eat. They are one of the nuts with the most nutrients, they contain 86% manganese, vitamins B1 and B6 as well as vitamin E and magnesium. They act as a powerful antioxidant and vasodilator. Consuming hazelnuts on a regular basis can reduce your risk of suffering from cardiovascular issues.

- Chestnuts: are unquestionably the nut with the highest starch content. Meaning, they contain the most carbohydrates and they are not very nutrient rich. They also don't contain much fat so they are the least recommended nut option.

- Walnuts, macadamia nuts, Brazil nuts and pecans: there is a lot of variety here. Depending on their origin, they vary in shape and size but they all share one thing and that is their high caloric content, making them one of the best fats in existence. They are also low in carbohydrates making them ideal to consume on a regular basis. Another wonderful thing about these nuts is that they have a good balance of omega-3 fatty acids and omega-6s, especially macadamia nuts. These kinds of nuts supply us many vitamins, minerals and antioxidants.

- Pine nuts: the kings of manganese and also low in carbohydrates. They are often used in Italian cuisine (essential in pesto sauce). The downside of this nut is that it can cause 'cacogeusia' otherwise known as pine mouth syndrome which basically is an unpleasurable, often times bitter or metallic aftertaste that can temporarily alter your sense of taste.

- Pistachios: originally from the Middle East and, unlike other nuts, generally found with a shell. They supply us with vitamins B1 and 6, phosphorus and other minerals – good for when we are working out.

DAIRY

Dairy is a grey area when it comes to our diet. Over the last 12,000 years our body has developed the ability to tolerate it. If this is true for you and you don't suffer from any digestive issues after consuming it and the dairy you consume comes from grass-fed cows then, it can be very beneficial to your health, such is the case with butter [Fig. 5].

'Dairy' is the word used when referring to all products made or derived from milk; yogurt, butter, and cream to name just a few.

The nutritional value and benefits of dairy are highly controversial and there is still a hot debate among supporters of the Paleo diet because science has not provided us with a solid answer as to whether dairy products are good or bad. However, the reality is that we have to go beyond that and not just focus on lists of what foods are allowed or prohibited. We have to listen to our body and do what suits us individually.

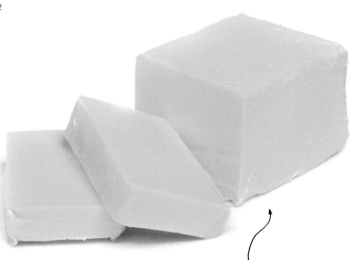

When organic, dairy is very healthy.

One of the main oppositions to dairy is that most people don't tolerate it well and that is because one of the main components in milk is lactose, which is milk sugar. In order to properly digest lactose, we need an enzyme called lactase which is produced in the small intestine. Well, if our body does not produce this enzyme or if it doesn't produce enough of it then our body cannot properly process dairy, resulting in discomfort, pain or just a simple intolerance to it.

Now, for people who are capable of producing lactase, dairy – when organic meaning from grass-fed cows, and consumed whole, that is

BUTTER VS. MARGARINE

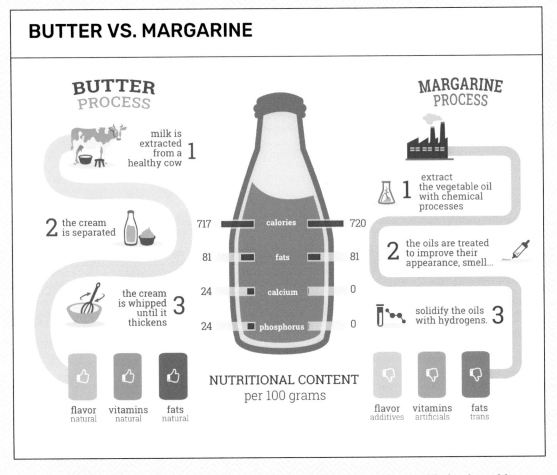

BUTTER PROCESS

milk is extracted from a healthy cow 1

2 the cream is separated

the cream is whipped until it thickens 3

flavor
natural

vitamins
natural

fats
natural

MARGARINE PROCESS

extract the vegetable oil with chemical processes 1

2 the oils are treated to improve their appearance, smell...

solidify the oils with hydrogens. 3

flavor
additives

vitamins
artificials

fats
trans

717	calories	720
81	fats	81
24	calcium	0
24	phosphorus	0

NUTRITIONAL CONTENT
per 100 grams

Figure 5: Butter from a healthy grass-fed cow is a natural product that supplies us with vitamins and fats. Margarine, on the other hand, is a product that can only be obtained through a chemical process.

to say not skimmed – is very healthy, rich in nutrients and is a good source of soluble vitamins and linoleic acid. These can help reduce the risk of disease and when fermented, they are rich in probiotics (good bacteria for our body's gastrointestinal health).

Depending on each individual's tolerance level, dairy can be consumed with caution while always making sure to find the highest quality product available. For example, butter is a very high-quality, very healthy fat, and a good source of omega-3 acids as well as vitamin K2. However, if you are someone who is lactose intolerant, or if you suffer from any autoimmune disease then it is best to avoid dairy and get medical supervision in order to avoid aggravating your condition further.

We can consume dairy cautiously, but always make sure it is of the highest quality.

I personally don't drink milk very often, but I do eat grass-fed butter, whole Greek yogurt, cream and sour cream from time to time.

I also occasionally eat matured cheeses like parmesan, fresh burrata or mozzarella, and I really like the creamy cheeses from the Swiss Alps which are made naturally from raw milk.

In short, is dairy Paleo? Well, that depends who you ask. My recommendation is to listen to your body, and do what it tells you, both with dairy and any other food.

LEGUMES

Legumes include peas, white and black beans, lentils, chickpeas, soybeans and products like miso or tofu which are derived from soybeans and so on.

While it is true that they contain natural fats and many minerals – among which iron stands out – they also contain high amounts of carbohydrates.

They are famous for causing gas, reflux and heartburn so it is important that we are prepared to digest them correctly.

As we saw with dairy, legumes are not suitable for everyone. Again, it depends on each individual. I myself hardly eat them which is not to say that they aren't part of my diet now and then.

NATURAL SWEETENERS

Most people love something sweet. Sweet flavours are pleasant and are culturally linked with leisure and enjoyment. The problem is that most desserts, sweets, snacks, ready-made drinks and processed foods contain alarming amounts of refined sugars, which as we know are very harmful to our health. In reality, almost every food we eat contains some kind of sugar, even if we aren't aware of it.

Living a natural lifestyle and avoiding refined sugar doesn't mean we have to give up that sweet taste. Many people believe that anything sweet makes you fat, and therefore to be healthy we have to set them aside. Luckily, there are several natural sweeteners you can use to make a variety of recipes, giving you the ability to cut out refined sugar from your diet while still enjoying something sweet. The best ones are:

- Raw honey: meaning not processed. It is a wonderful natural food. This honey is pure, no additives and you can get it in powder or liquid form. Honey contains many nutrients such as sodium, potassium, magnesium, iron and vitamins A, C and B in addition to glucose AND it is a natural carbohydrate.

- Stevia: This is the only natural sweetener that is calorie-free. It is perfect for anyone with diabetes or those who want to lose weight. The leaf can be eaten fresh, dried or in powder form. Although powdered stevia is processed, all they really do is dry the leaf and grind it. It is great to use in drinks.

Stevia has been used by Paraguayans for 1,500 years.

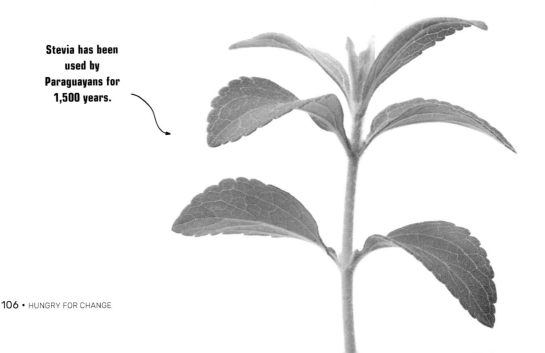

- Maple syrup: is the natural sap from a variety of different maple species. It is a 100% natural plant product, making it suitable for vegetarians and vegans. It is a fantastic sweetener for desserts.

- Molasses and panela: both come from the natural syrup that is naturally extracted from sugar cane, and can be in liquid or solid form. An important thing to keep in mind is that its flavour can be somewhat more intense than the other sweeteners on our list and its dark colour is not always appetising. Even so, you can enjoy this completely natural sweetener by adjusting the proportions you use.

Processed products: desserts, sweets, snacks and beverages contain alarming amounts of refined sugars that are very harmful to our health.

- Coconut sugar: is the perfect alternative to replace sugar in any recipe, since it is granulated and closely resembles table sugar. The sweetness is also just about the same, so you don't have to worry about calculating different proportions. Its main benefit is its low glycemic index.

BE CAREFUL WITH SUGAR

In general, we should consume sugars in moderation, even those that are naturally present in fruits, honey, and maple syrup. Although it is natural sugar (whether it is refined or not) the way it is processed in the body is the same, and therefore, if we over-consume it, we can cause ourselves to have a hormonal imbalance and possibly become insulin resistant.

FOODS TO AVOID IN OUR DIET

Most cereals contain gluten (a protein that is present in wheat, barley, rye. It is what makes the dough elastic) and other antinutrients, such as lectin (a protein that is also found in legumes), which makes digestion difficult and can cause many people's intestines to become inflamed.

Cereals contain large amounts of carbohydrates which are then transformed into glucose when consumed. We eat far more carbohydrates today then our ancestors could even imagine almost three million years ago, as they didn't even begin to grow them until the agrarian revolution during the Neolithic era.

The foods we must avoid at all costs are those that are ultra-processed. Unfortunately, that means most of what we find in the supermarket today. Ultra-processed foods are made through industrial procedures and contain large amounts of artificial additives. Usually, these products last a long time compared to their natural counterparts. The industry also uses colourants and flavouring in these products to make them more attractive and appetising to consumers.

Behind their seemingly harmless appearance, these are highly dangerous foods. Why? Because they are full of hidden trans fats, all kinds of sugars, artificial additives and, vegetable oils, whose origins are often unknown. Moreover, they lack nutritional value and what little they might offer only comes in the form of artificially added' vitamins' and 'minerals'.

IT IS EASIER THAN YOU THINK TO SUBSTITUTE THESE FOODS

Wheats, juices, oils and sugar — we already know that the food industry has greatly transformed these products by creating genetically modified versions, whose final product barely resembles the original. Besides the addition of enormous amounts of refined sugars, and/or chemicals, the process itself of how they handle these foods greatly reduces their nutritional quality. This means that the usable calories from artificial products are significantly lower than those provided by their natural alternative. As a result, we end up eating foods that are harmful to our health.

Additionally, we should also not abuse certain natural foods as that is also not good for our health. Gluten and lectins that are naturally found in cereals and legumes, or starch which is naturally present in potatoes, are all elements that are hard for our body to process correctly, making it difficult for our digestive system to function properly.

The good news is that there are countless numbers of natural alternatives to all the foods that don't help us develop and that aren't beneficial to our health. Below is a short list of just some of the options available, which we hope will get your imagination flowing:

Ultra-processed food	Natural alternative
refined sugar, artificial sweeteners	dates, raisins, coconut sugar, honey
refined wheat flour	almond flour, quinoa flour, buckwheat flour
lactose-free milk	plant-based milks: coconut, almond, walnut
bottled juices	homemade smoothies
sunflower oil, corn oil	virgin olive oil, almond oil, avocado oil, butter
margarine	butter, avocado
white bread	dried fruits (walnuts, hazelnuts, cashews, pistachios, pine nuts...)
noodles, spaghetti	courgetti (strips of courgette), strips of carrots or squid
French fries	oven-baked veggie chips
rice, legumes	quinoa, amaranth, or grated cauliflower
potato	sweet potato

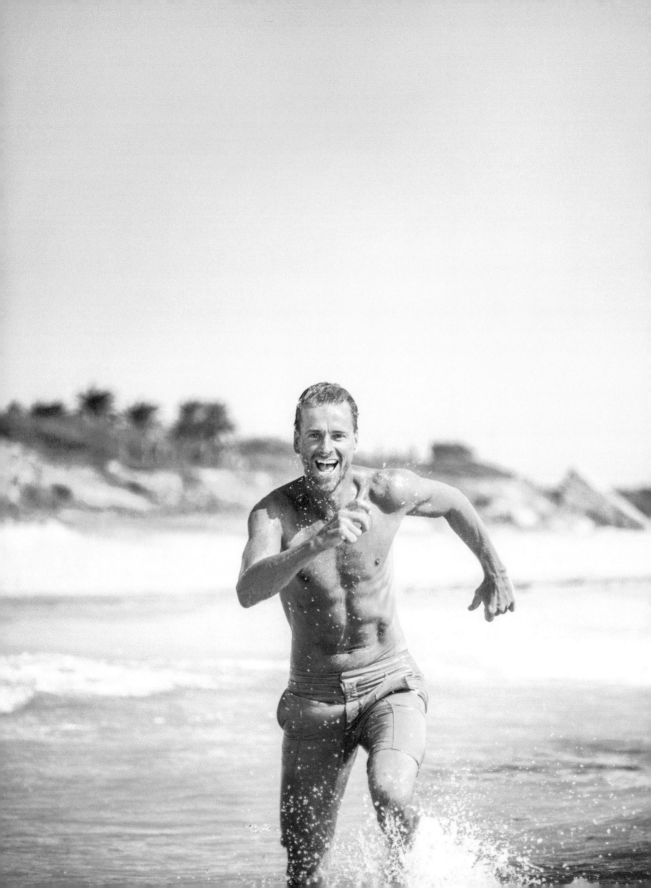

THE IMPORTANCE
OF EXERCISE

DESPITE EVERYTHING AT OUR DISPOSAL these days, society has never been so physically inactive as now. Before, being active was a necessary part of a human's life. However, nowadays, if we do exercise it is done as a social act and even in some cases it is done as something trendy. We have 'unlearned' how to exercise. What's worse is that we have abandoned our own body's natural movements. Luckily though, we still have the power to move our body in the same way our ancestors did.

Office work, being a couch potato, electric scooters, online entertainment – there are many reasons why people aren't exercising. Although working out may seem trendy, percentage-wise not many people are. And those who do are often just trying to burn off that excess energy that they've consumed through their poor diets rather than thinking about the other benefits that come from exercising.

We often associate exercise with playing sports or doing intense work outs and often falsely believe that only a privileged few can do so. These are all misconceptions and excuses. We don't need to run 10km every day or go out every morning on our mountain bike to be active. Just breaking our daily sedentary routine is enough. Go for a walk, take the stairs instead of the lift, do those small things that make your heart and body work just a little more than it usually does.

Exercise (not just sport) is important for both our physical and mental well-being. It not only makes us feel better but it makes us smarter.

BRAIN FUNCTION AND EXERCISE GO HAND IN HAND

Physical exercise makes our blood circulate rapidly throughout our body and not just in the areas we are moving but it also activates the blood flow to our brain. This is in essence what feeds our brain, giving it more nutrients, stimulating its plasticity and encouraging the growth of new neurons. Exercising does all this and more:

- **Improves mental health:** various scientific studies have shown that physical exercise can restore neurotransmitters (our brains' messengers) such as glutamate and GABA which decrease when we are depressed. This is why physical activity makes us feel better and is often used as a treatment for serious illnesses such as depression.

- **Reduces the risk of dementia:** regular physical activity improves the overall cognitive skills of people suffering from Alzheimer's. It has also been proven that senior citizens who don't have Alzheimer's but are physically active are significantly less likely to develop the disease compared to their sedentary counterparts.

- **Increases brain plasticity:** brain plasticity is an essential part of our nervous system and is what allows us to grow and adapt throughout our lives. Physical exercise allows us to enhance this. Continual aerobic physical exercise stimulates neuro-genesis, which is the creation of neurons in the hippocampus, a fundamental area of our brain responsible for learning and memory.

- **Keeps stress at bay:** it has been scientifically proven that physical activity causes the brain to respond less to stress and keeps anxiety from interfering in our daily lives. In other words, physical exercise creates a mental state where we are able to respond more appropriately to stressful stimuli that we are subjected to in our daily lives.

HOW MUCH DO YOU HAVE TO EXERCISE TO GET ALL THESE BENEFITS?

The amount of exercise required depends on many factors, but the simplest way to group it is by age:

- **Children and teenagers between the ages of 5 and 17** should spend at least 60 minutes a day doing moderate to intense physical activities (sports, physical education etc.). The majority of their daily physical activity should be aerobic.

- **Adults (18+)** should spend at least 150 minutes a week doing some kind of moderate to intense aerobic physical activity, or 75 minutes of vigorous aerobic physical activity, breaking sessions into no less than 10-minute segments. This can be going for walk, riding a bike, doing chores, playing sports etc. Of course, the longer you do per week the more benefits you'll gain.

THE INCENTIVES AND REWARDS OF PLAYING SPORTS

The brain's design is so complex that in addition to giving us the physical gratification both during and after exercising it also releases certain hormones that push us to go further and harder even when we think we are too tired to continue.

Suddenly, something stimulates our motor system and pushes us to continue on. It is something you can only experience when you push your physical body to the limit. It is what has allowed us to survive.

This is that flight or fight mode when our body feels the need to stay alert. In those moments our brain sends an order to our endocrine system to release a hormone called adrenaline.

Adrenaline increases muscle tension, blood pressure, blood glucose levels and the rate at which our brain neurons fire. These biological alterations make us think, act and, react more quickly, resulting in higher productivity.

Adrenaline does more than that: even low-intensity exercise or aerobic exercise positively affect our brain. It improves our capacity to reason, improves creativity and helps improve our memory. Adrenaline awakens our brain and activates our nerve cells.

Don't forget: exercise is good for your body and mind.

You may also have heard that exercising is addictive; that feeling can be attributed to the hormone dopamine that the body releases during physical activity. Stimulants, drugs, and sugary foods all trigger the same release of dopamine into the blood stream. It gives us a feeling of pleasure and euphoria. That effect is what makes us want to do something over and over again.

As I just mentioned, exercise does the same thing. The brain orders the endocrine system to release a small dose of dopamine into the blood. This is what explains the feeling of joy, happiness and relaxation that we experience after we exercise. This is why people say sport is like a drug. Once you're hooked you can't stop.

What's more, there is also a substance in our body called serotonin that amplifies the positive effect that we receive from dopamine. Known as the hormone of happiness, serotonin regulates our mood, sleep and appetite.

Physical activity is one way we increase the tryptophan levels in our body, which is a great precursor to the release of serotonin. The release of serotonin motivates us and gives us a feeling of well-being and joy.

Our brain is also capable of alleviating the sensation of pain when we work out, by releasing endorphins. These hormones work like morphine. They help alleviate pain by increasing the feeling of well-being, and allow us to prolong the duration of our work-out even if we have suffered an injury. This is precisely why when we stop our activity the pain comes back or feels more intense, because the release of endorphins has stopped.

As you can see, there are many benefits to being physically active, not only for the body but for the mind as well.

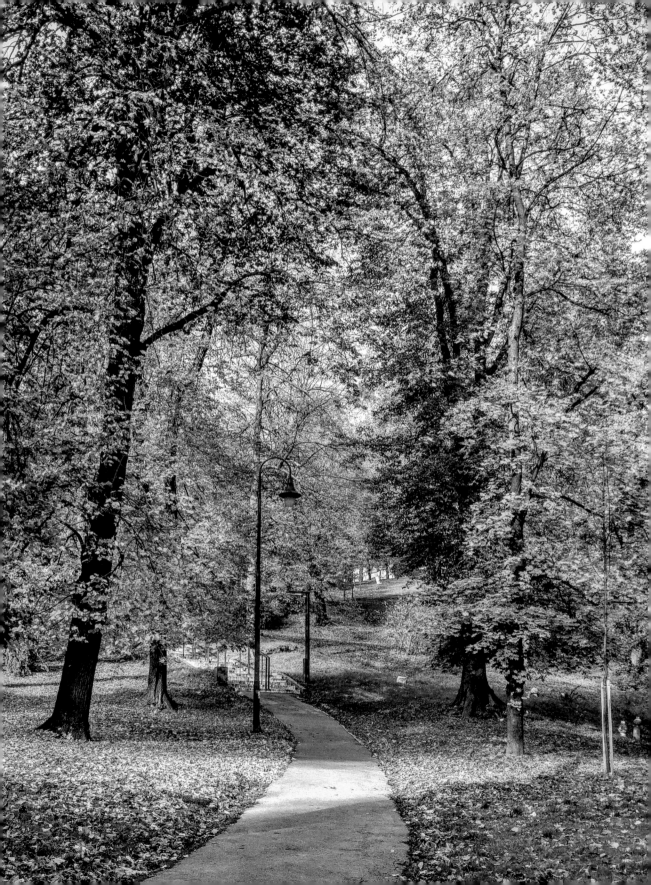

SLEEP AND REST

WE SPEND A THIRD of our lives sleeping, which averages out to about seven to eight hours a night. However, I very much doubt that the young generation of today spend a third of their lives sleeping, because of the evolution of technology. This new age has had a negative impact on the amount and quality of sleep we are getting. For instance, research shows that the exposure to artificial light through our devices disrupts our sleep patterns. This combined with a bad diet has greatly influenced how much and what kind of sleep we are getting.

Sleep is necessary in order to 'reset' our body both physically and mentally. It is as vital to our body as water or eating. In the 1960s the average American adult slept about eight and half hours a day. Since then, the percentage has only declined: in 1998 only 35% of American adults slept eight hours a day and in 2005 only 26% did. Today with the improvements of living conditions we should be focused on recovering the length of time we sleep and the quality of that sleep.

Sadly though, these days the average adult sleeps around six and a half hours a night, which has serious health consequences and negatively affects our quality of life. These negative effects aren't

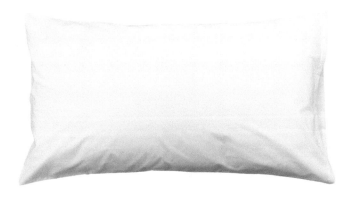

just weight gain but, people who sleep fewer than eight hours a day are also more predisposed to type 2 diabetes, or suffering from insulin-resistance or sleep hormone imbalances, as well as other hormonal imbalances related to appetite and the feeling of being full.

In one clinical study they researched the connection between getting 4 hours of sleep and the effect on hormones that are responsible for our appetite and satiety (ghrelin and leptin). They observed that there was a 24% drop in overall satiety and a 32% increase in appetite. Interestingly, the increase in appetite was for products that are rich in sugar, such as chocolates or cookies. And that's not all, another study showed when people who only slept 4 hours were given a choice between healthy food and junk food their brain was more stimulated when they were offered the latter. Ultimately both studies found that the less sleep we get the hungrier we are, for junk food that is (Taheri et al. 2004).

BUT HOW DOES SLEEP WORK?

Our sleep cycle is divided into two major phases. During the first phase, our brain waves are faster and more frequent, and there is some muscle activity and rapid eye movement. During the second phase there is an absence of muscle activity and eye movement combined with slower brain waves. When you sleep for the recommended 8 hours a night, you go through between four and five cycles that last between 90 and 120 minutes and these can be divided into five stages:

- **Stage 1:** light sleep. This is the first phase that we already mentioned above, where rapid eye movement and some muscle spasms occur.

- **Stage 2:** the eyes no longer move and our brain waves slow down. This is when we enter the second stage that we mentioned previously.

- **Stages 3 and 4:** are the stages in which we sleep most soundly and are connected to the second sleep stage where our brain waves move slowly.

- **Stage REM:** this is when our brain has a registered activity that is more similar to those we have during the day (wakefulness); that is because this is the stage where dreams occur.

Melatonin is the hormone regulating this sleep cycle. It is synthesised from the amino acid tryptophan. This hormone synchronises the body's natural cycle of sleep and wakefulness. It also decreases body temperature. A finely regulated melatonin cycle can be altered by an excess of a stress hormone called cortisol.

Cortisol created naturally assists the sleep cycle. It is often known as the body's natural alarm clock. With concentrations of the hormone peaking during the day and lowering at night, it promotes the production of melatonin during the sleep cycle. However, cortisol levels can increase when subjected to stress, which negatively affects our rest. It produces a state of alertness within our body and causes insomnia, making it difficult for a person to fall asleep.

It is advisable to include foods rich in tryptophan at dinner to improve the production of melatonin, which facilitates better quality sleep.

Food has a lot to do with having a properly functioning sleep cycle. In fact, there are certain foods that are considered to be sleep-inducing thanks to their high concentration of tryptophan (the amino acid precursor to melatonin). This is why it would make sense to try and include them in your dinner, thus promoting an improved production of melatonin, resulting in better sleep.

Some examples of food that are rich in tryptophan and offer great nutritional value are pumpkin, sunflower seeds and sesame seeds. The last have a high concentration of omega-6 acids as well as very good anti-inflammatory properties which greatly improve the quality of your sleep. Tuna also has a lot of tryptophan and omega-3. Cheese and beef are also rich in this amino acid which again is the precursor to the production of melatonin.

While a good diet and one rich in tryptophan helps, it is not the only factor in solving the problem of sleep. So, what else should we do? Well, the answer is quite simple: get back to healthy patterns and sleep routines.

Here are some tips for getting a restful night's sleep, which we all need.

- Reduce your exposure to artificial light such as that from electronic devices. Remember, television also emits blue light which keeps us from falling asleep. This light actually decreases the production of melatonin!

- Go to bed early and stop watching TV, checking your emails, and chatting on your phone at least two hours before going to bed. Our sleep is controlled by different hormones that follow a 24-hour cycle. Respecting this will help us to fall asleep faster and improve our quality of sleep.

- Switch to an analogue alarm clock. If you can't live without your digital alarm clock then cover it with a cloth at night to prevent the light from coming through.

- Keep the room dark by using blackout curtains or blinds.

- Turn off any mobile device or activate the 'sleep mode' if it has one. This will stop email notifications and other kinds of notifications from coming through and interrupting you while you sleep.

- A good trick to use on those days when you are sleeping away from home is to use a sleep mask. That way you can make sure that no light rays are disturbing your restful sleep.

- Don't go to bed hungry or too full. Centennials often say that to live longer you should eat until you feel comfortable. In fact, there is a saying in Japan that says, 'one should eat until they are 60-70% satiated'.

Sesame seeds are rich in tryptophan and promote and encourage a good night's sleep.

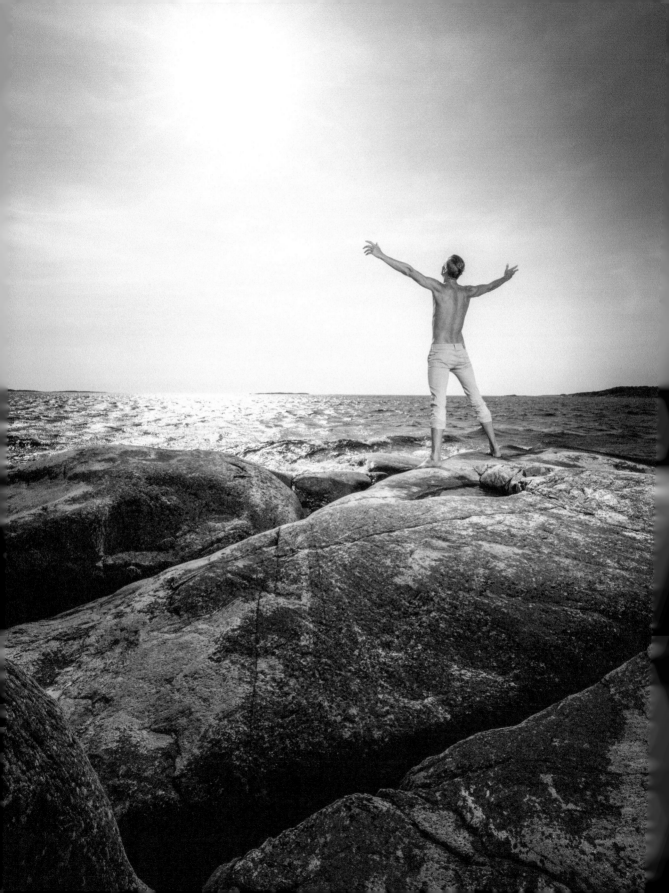

THE SUN AND
FRESH AIR

THANKS TO THE SUN, LIFE is possible on our planet. The vast majority of living things need the sun to survive and humans are no exception.

Moderate sun exposure has great health benefits, since it activates our metabolism, and positively affects our mood. Our bodies have always been exposed to sun naturally as our ancestors were nomads. They would have to move from one place to another, walking long hours during the day under the heat of the sun.

Due to climate change and the damage we have inflicted on nature over the last several centuries, the ozone layer has got thinner and thinner – in some parts of the world it has become almost non-existent – so we have to be careful with ultraviolet rays and protect ourselves.

Although the sun has many benefits, let's not forget that an excess of sun exposure can be very damaging to our health, causing sunburn, premature ageing (to the most exposed areas, face, neck and hands), dehydration, headaches, fatigue, dizziness and eventually skin cancer.

This is why it is so important to take care of ourselves when we are in the sun and protect our skin at all times – not just when we are tanning on the beach but any time we are going to be exposed.

In spite of all that, the sun is our first and greatest source of energy and the driving factor of the existence of life on earth. Its light and heat provide us with incredible health benefits; by just going for a bike ride, or run and even just a walk in the sun you can activate your body. Take a look at the list of all the positive benefits that sunlight has on our health:

- **Increases Serotonin levels:** the sun has been proven to increase the amount of Serotonin in the body. This hormone is very important as it helps with proper digestion, balances out our mood, controls body temperature, influences our sexual desires, reduces aggressiveness and helps to regulate our sleep cycles.

- **Improves the condition of our skin:** a little sunbathing can be very beneficial for those with acne, psoriasis or jaundice. Remember not to overdo it, 10 to 20 minutes at the beginning or end of the day when the sunrays are not as strong is more than enough. Always use sunscreen, never wait for your skin to start getting red before putting some on as it is a clear sign that you've already been burned.

- **Helps our immune system:** the sun increases the level of white blood cells in our blood, which are responsible for executing an immune response to attacks on our body from foreign substances and antigens that cause infections and other ailments.

- **Strengthens our teeth and bone tissue:** the sun's rays trigger the production of vitamin D in our body. Unlike other vitamins that we can obtain through food, our skin generates vitamin D when it is stimulated by the sun. This vitamin helps us to absorb calcium and phosphorus which both help to strengthen bones. In Nordic countries, where the sun is often hidden behind the cloud, people often take vitamin D supplements from birth.

- **Helps lower blood pressure:** the sun's rays can also help to reduce blood pressure, as one of its positive benefits is its effectiveness as a vasodilator. In addition, by activating our metabolism it also allows more tissue to be cleansed.

The sun isn't the only thing that benefits us, different studies have shown that people who live near green landscapes have a lower risk of suffering from respiratory and cardiovascular diseases. The simple fact is that being surrounded by nature gives us a sense of peace. And although ultimately our diet is the most important and influential factor in our lives, the activities we do should also be based on the same principles. A connection to the outdoors and nature has many great advantages:

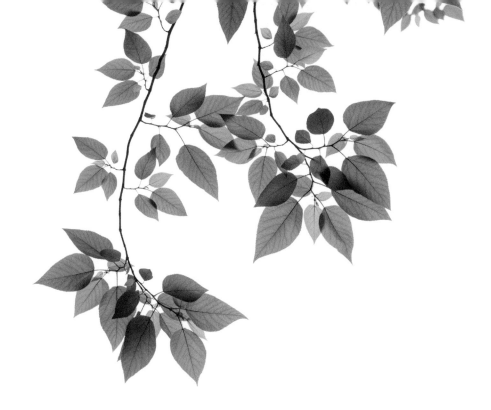

- **Being connected to nature reduces stress:** when we feel better, our body reduces the amount of cortisol (the stress hormone) that it releases. Several studies have shown that walking through green landscapes changes our brain activity by reducing stress and cortisol levels as well as blood pressure.

- **Being outdoors encourages physical activity:** many people find it much more enjoyable to go for a walk, run, climb or bike ride outside as it is infinitely better to exercise recreationally than being confined to the four walls of a gym.

- **It oxygenates us:** the air quality in natural spaces outside city limits is much higher. It's a truism, but many times we don't stop and think about how stale the air inside our homes and workplaces is, and how harmful it can be in the long run.

In short, being connected to nature in our daily lives reduces our chances of dying from cardiovascular or respiratory diseases such as asthma. That is because it drives us to be more active, feel more relaxed and we get the necessary vitamin D for our body to thrive.

INTERMITTENT FASTING

HUMANS are physically prepared to go through periods of fasting as we were forced to for thousands of years due to the limited food availability. In fact, most doctors agree that the body can survive without food for up to eight weeks. During a fasting period, many processes are altered within the body – for example, our hormones and restorative capabilities change. During a fast our body's insulin levels decrease which reverses the fat-storing process and in the long run helps to prevent cardiovascular disease and chronic diseases such as diabetes.

During the fast you can consume any type of broth, infusions or teas.

I learned about the benefits of fasting and the various ways to fast for many years. Some of my friends fasted on maple syrup mixes and others on different kinds of syrup. However, after studying the subject in depth, I respectfully am of the opinion that this type of fast does not get you the benefits that come with a true fast. This means that only water, tea, or black coffee should be consumed rather than anything that contains sugar or other calories.

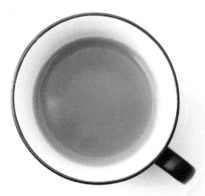

What surprised me most when I began to fast was my energy level. I fast a couple of times or more each month. I eat a good dinner of protein and fat while trying to eat as little carbs as possible. Afterwards, I begin my 24-hour countdown.

I don't eat anything for breakfast, I only have a cup of tea with some almond milk. Between 10am and 2pm I usually feel a bit hungry but I avoid eating anything and just stick to drinking water. The feeling usually goes away around 2pm and I feel good until dinner time. The strange part is that even when I work out these days without having eaten anything, I still have more energy than I usually would on any other day. After my 24 hours of fasting, I eat dinner and of course I have a very good appetite by that time and although I eat more, I don't overdo it – I'm not eating three times the amount I should. I don't recommend fasting for children, women who are pregnant or for anyone who suffers from any sort of disease. However, if that is not your case than I highly suggest you try it and see the results for yourself.

Fasting promotes the growth and production of hormones, helps burns fat, stimulates muscle development and delays ageing.

Fasting is known to promote the growth and production of hormones, help burn more fat, stimulate muscle development, delay ageing and reduce inflammation in the body.

When you fast, your sugar and blood insulin levels drop drastically. Fasting also reduces the production of ghrelin (the hunger hormone), so we are better able to control our appetite throughout the day.

Various studies have also shown that fasting helps limit the growth of cancer cells and improves cholesterol levels. It's also been proven to have positive effects on the brain by improving self-control. Many times, we think we are hungry when in reality we are not. So, by overcoming we become more self-disciplined and regulated. It's like when you run long distance, after 3 kilometres you feel tired but you are able to push through and run twice that. Our mind is simply trained to tell us 'that's fine now'.

FOOD
SUSTAINABILITY

A RESPECT FOR NATURE is part of living a natural lifestyle, which is why it is important to consume products that come from farms that use the most natural procedures and techniques possible when caring for their livestock, orchards, or crops. This means respecting seasonal growth and the environment at all times.

Agriculture and livestock produce about 20% of greenhouse gas emissions and use about 80% of land used by man. Massive cereal and vegetable crops to feed livestock have led to the deforestation of many places.

That is why it is essential to find a balance between consuming local and easy-to-obtain (thanks to globalisation) foreign goods. In other words, we should always try to consume seasonal products from places that are as close to us as possible, whenever feasible. That way we avoid further impacting the environment with the transportation of these goods.

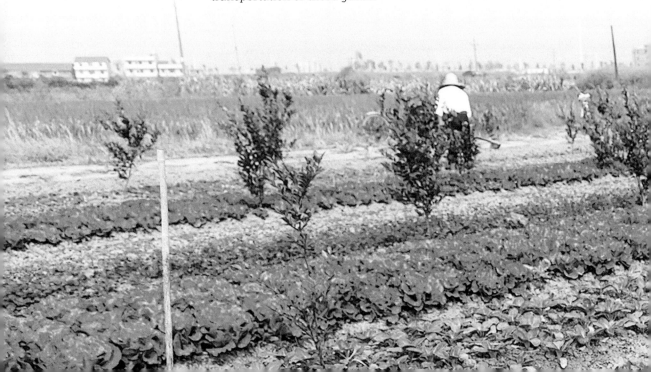

To take a personal example from my adopted country: while not all climates make it possible to have food diversity throughout the year, Spain does. We are lucky, as Spain has a large diversity of local natural products throughout the year. We just have to adapt to what nature provides us each season.

Lluís Serra-Majem, a professor of Preventive Medicine and Public Health at the University of Las Palmas de Gran Canaria, summarises the challenge of doing this in four parts (Serra-Majem 2010):

- Integrate biological and ecological methods and processes in food production.

- Minimise the use of non-renewable substrates that damage our environment and as a consequence, our health.

- Make more efficient and better use of knowledge and techniques from farmers.

- Work together as a team in order to solve problems such as intensive farming.

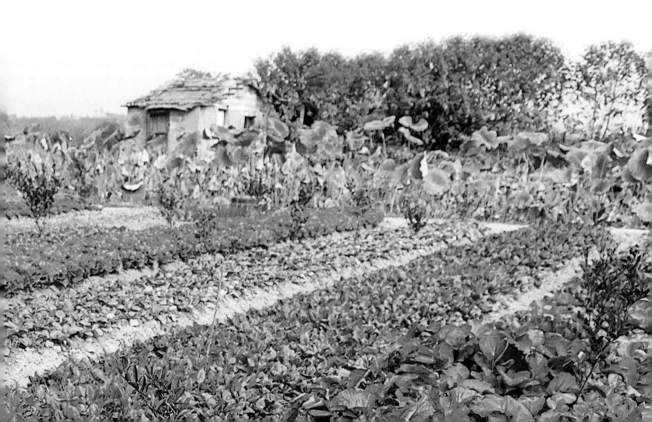

A NATURAL DIET
FOR CHILDREN

PROVIDING A NATURAL DIET to children is not only possible but necessary. It is vital that they receive all the necessary nutrients, vitamins and minerals they need to grow healthy and strong and at the same time be protected from the damage caused by eating poorly, as unfortunately many adults have done. Children are 'cleaner' and so by feeding them a natural diet they will reap even more of the benefits.

It is important to start doing this as soon as possible, as they should start learning about good eating habits from a young age. During childhood is when we learn and form our own habits that often will last us a lifetime, like for example, brushing your teeth, making your bed, and even being active.

If from a young age, we instill in our children the importance of good nutrition and expose them to healthy foods, then we will ensure that they will continue to follow these healthy habits into adulthood. If on the other hand, we get them used to a poor diet, one that includes processed foods and is rich in sugar and refined carbohydrates, then we aren't giving them a good foundation for a healthy future.

That isn't to say though that we should forbid all of these foods, as this will only make them want them more. It's best to offer them healthy alternatives that taste naturally sweet and pleasant but that don't contain refined sugars. This teaches them that tasty doesn't have to mean junk.

Regardless, there are several factors that play against us as parents when it comes to feeding our children a healthy natural diet, which is why Spain tops the list for most obese children in Europe.

Nowadays we have quick and easy access to food, we also have an excessive amount of processed food options such as biscuits, fizzy drinks, doughnuts you name it... However, what may be worse still is the general misinformation that children are being taught when it comes to nutrition and food. They are still being taught in school the 'traditional food pyramid' where flour, cereals and potatoes are considered more important than fruits and vegetables!

Another problem is that we are used to rewarding our children with junk. Let's face it; a child never gets rewarded with an apple - most opt for a chocolate bar, maybe an ice cream, or a trip to a fast-food joint for a hamburger. So, what happens when we do this? Well, we get children used to associating feeling good with consuming junk. Of course, we want children to enjoy food and enjoy eating – however, many adolescents and adults develop eating disorders that lead them to binge when they are sad or stressed because they've learned from a young age that this food makes them feel good and they feel comforted by it; thus, harming them even further.

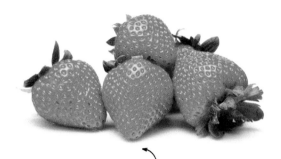

Why don't we reward our children with some delicious strawberries instead of with sweets?

Which leads me to my next point; don't underestimate the impact of advertising. There are so many ads that are exclusively designed to target children. Ones for chocolate milk that make you the best, others for cookies that give you energy and even yogurts with superpowers. All of which just entice your children more and put more pressure on the 'need' to have these things.

A very common question to ask is whether eating healthy is worthwhile. Many parents see healthy food as more expensive than unhealthy foods which leads to many occasions where the reason for buying a particular food isn't its nutritional quality but rather its price. But here's the dilemma: don't we want our children to have the best? Don't we want them to grow up strong and healthy? The cost of a quality diet is more than justified. The money we spend on a natural diet for our children is one of the best future investments we can make. There is no better investment than in your children's health.

With that said, it is true that often times children simply refuse to eat things like vegetables because they don't like them. This is partly caused by the bitter taste that many veggies have due to their high calcium content. Green veggies such as broccoli, chard, cabbage, and onions are great sources of calcium but, eating them on their own can be unpleasant. So, it's a good idea to combine these foods with others like tomatoes, meats, eggs, quinoa, and

A snack bar made with dates, nuts and chia is all-natural and an ideal snack for kids.

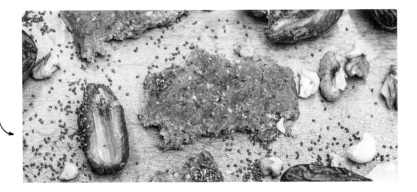

sweet potatoes in order to almost hide them from your children. Making a nice puree or stew is one way to do this.

Another great trick to get your children to want to eat more vegetables is to let them choose. Not only are they happier because they are eating something they have chosen, but they also are then able to gradually cultivate their own interest in natural foods. The same goes for fish. When you involve your children in the purchasing and preparation process, they become more motivated and interested in eating what they've helped to make.

Despite some of the obvious drawbacks to doing all of this, (longer cooking times, making sure your child doesn't always choose the same thing etc.) we should remember that everything a child learns during their formative years, especially those first years of life, is imprinted in their brain and they will continue to repeat these things throughout their life subconsciously.

In my personal case, my children started eating this way a couple years ago and speaking from my own experience, not only are they in perfect health and growing, but they also love this new way of eating. They've even started rejecting processed foods on their own and have become authentically natural themselves.

Although at the beginning it may seem difficult, the process of switching from a conventional diet to a natural one for children is not that much different than that for adults, it might even be considered easier since children are probably more adaptable and flexible in terms of their habits.

In any case, it is a process that should be done progressively so that the change lasts over time. Remember that our goal is not to look for a magical recipe but rather to realise that our diet, a natural one, is the optimal fuel for our body to lead a healthy and active lifestyle.

My sons are 11 and 9 respectively and they at one point ate what was considered 'normal' amounts of sugar, and sweets for children and often times people tend to say 'they are kids, it's fine' but, it isn't fine. Things do happen when a child has a diet based on processed foods that are targeted specifically to them – cereals, yogurts, biscuits, fruit juice, the list goes on and at the end of the day the amount of sugar they've consumed is excessively high.

My children began to gradually change their habits meaning it didn't happen overnight, and as parents we have to be patient because this change can take time. Little by little they replaced their breakfast cereal with fruit and started to find alternatives to other foods until the majority of their diet was based on fruits and vegetables. On special occasions, like a birthday, we substituted store-bought ice cream for natural homemade ice cream without the added sugar instead. We also often make some fruit skewers as a sweet treat.

My children and I became healthier as a family, and not just physically but in other ways as well. Once we cut out the refined sugars and grains, I especially noticed a change in my children. They were able to concentrate better when doing their homework, they would fall asleep more easily and they went from being a bit hyperactive to more relaxed.

Interestingly enough, they usually refuse to eat processed foods now – they don't really enjoy them. A fundamental part of this change is because they were involved in the reasons behind the change and started to participate in the cooking process. For me personally, this is one of the many benefits I think a natural diet provides. There is no choice but to cook and prepare all the food you buy and that takes time, and that time can be spent as a family. I really take advantage of this quality bonding time. Of course, my children are not the same age and so naturally their responsibilities in the kitchen are different but they each can always participate.

Please, don't think that my children don't eat cookies or sweets, they do. However, they are homemade. There are countless natural recipes that are sugar-free and don't contain any grains and they are still delicious! One of their favourites is coconut and banana cookies.

I know this may all seem difficult, but I promise it isn't. It is only a matter of starting the process little by little. The change will come gradually and without you really realising it. It will improve many aspects of the whole family's life.

BEFORE
THE RECIPES

I've been writing my blog on Paleo for the past three years and what I've always enjoyed most is hearing the comments from people all over the world (Natruly Blog 2021). Messages such as: 'I've been following you for a few months, following your lifestyle advice, and I've lost weight, slept better, I work out more and just enjoy life more'. Comments like that are what excite me and keep me going. They are the ones which inspired me to write this book.

My goal with this book has been to share my experiences with you and to help others feel better.

After all, the most important thing is to enjoy life and spend time with the people you love.

You may have come across a lot of new information on how to lead a more natural lifestyle in this book and feel overwhelmed. You may be feeling like you would need to make too many changes, but don't worry. The important thing is if this book has awakened your interest in living a more natural and better life. To find the balance that makes you feel more positive, more comfortable and that allows you to be the best version of yourself. Because, after all, the most important thing is to enjoy the life with have with the ones we love.

This book is not meant to be a set of rules that you must start tomorrow and follow down to the 'T'. It is quite the opposite in fact. This book is rather some simple suggestions on how you can apply alternative methods and foods as you see fit and at your own pace. Each step you take towards living a more natural life will be tremendously beneficial to you and your family. Each small step in that direction makes the next one just that much easier.

And, don't worry about being too strict either. Even if you decide that rice doesn't suit you, does that mean you can't go and have sushi with friends?

Of course not! If the majority of the time you are leading a natural and healthy lifestyle and reaping those benefits, then slipping up or enjoying a treat every now and again isn't going to hurt you.

Last but certainly not least, I leave you with perhaps the most important piece of advice I can give:

BE SCEPTICAL

Be sceptical of everything, including this book. The food industry is one of the largest global industries and there are many conflicts of interest when it comes to profits and health. The best way to stay safe and protect our health is to be sceptical. Once you look into things for yourself and have the data, do what you think is most beneficial to your health. Be your own guide. Be sceptical of labels, product packaging, tv commercials, articles on nutrition in the newspaper... be sceptical about everything claimed regarding food.

Think about what you're being told and decide for yourself if the information fits. Find facts to back up what you think is good for you and act accordingly. If we all take the time and make the effort do this, we can change the world.

My own scepticism and enthusiasm to help others is what gave me the energy and led me to create Natruly with my business partner Octavio. We are going to have some interesting years ahead of us but I'm convinced that we are going to change the world.

Because changing what we eat is the first step to changing the world.

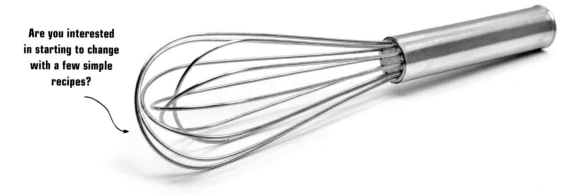

Are you interested in starting to change with a few simple recipes?

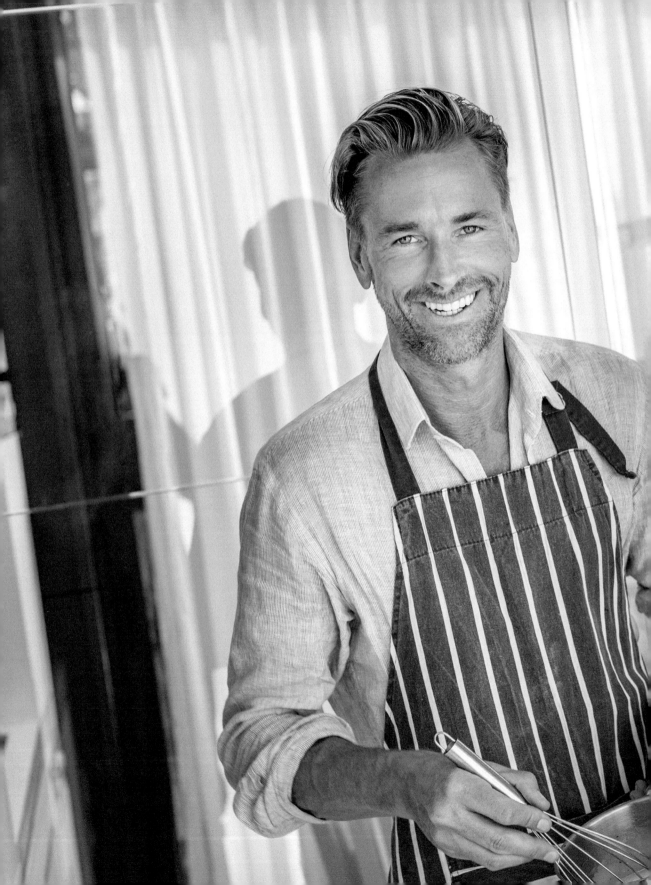

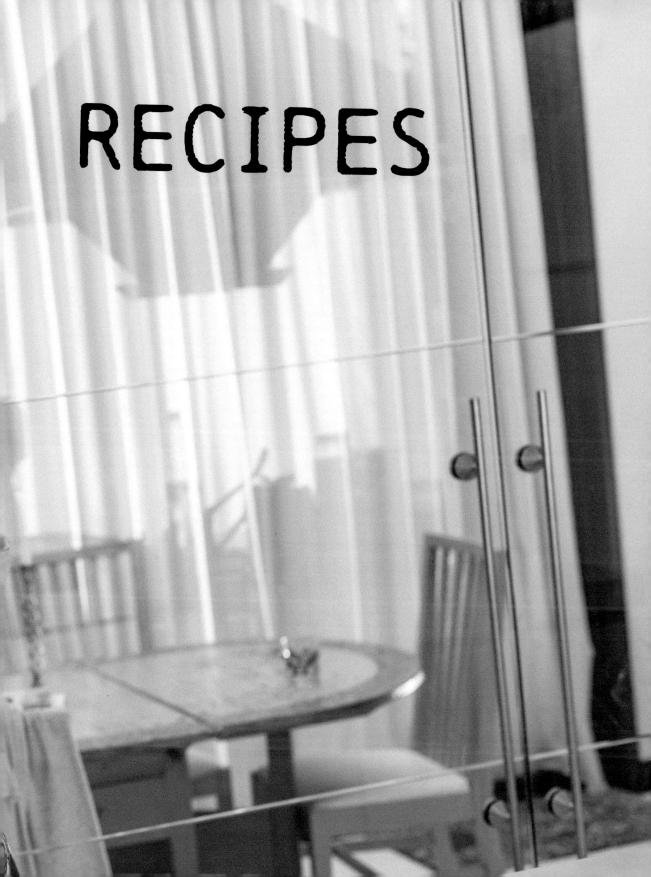

RECIPES

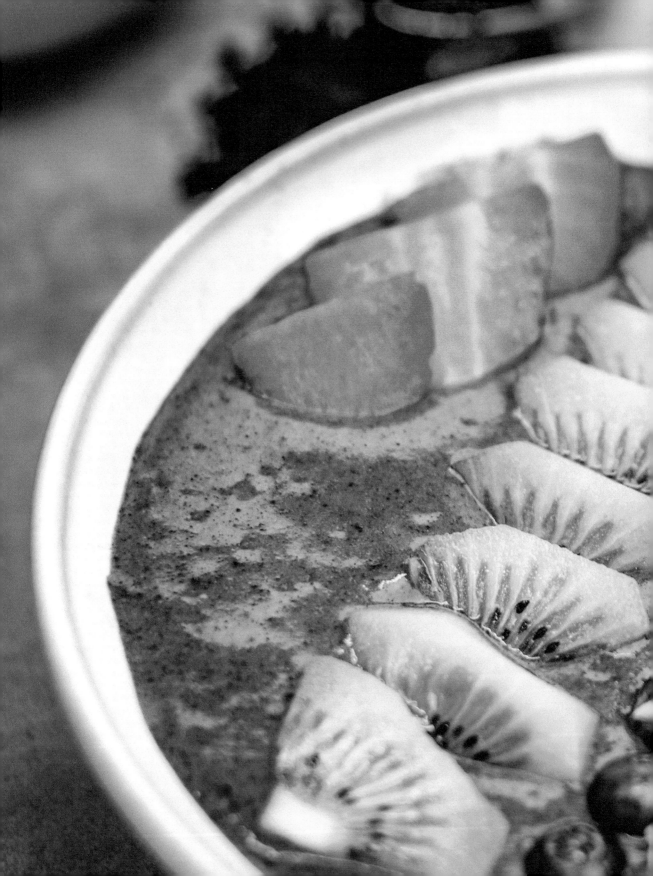

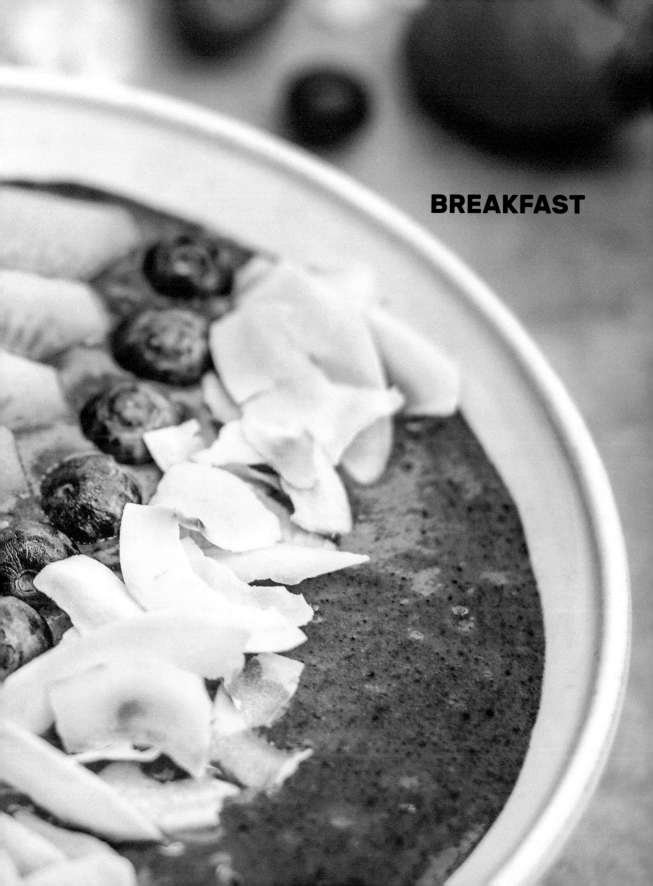

BREAKFAST

ASPARAGUS AND SHIITAKE MUSHROOM OMELETTE

♟ Serves: **2**

⏱ Time: **20 minutes**

INGREDIENTS

6 eggs

1 bundle of green asparagus

150g shiitake mushrooms

100g cabbage

salt and pepper

6 tbsps butter

UTENSILS

pan, spatula, knife

- Wash all the vegetables including the mushrooms well and then dice them into small pieces.

- Place 3 tbsps butter in your pan and sauté the vegetables and mushrooms for 5 minutes over medium heat.

- In a bowl, beat the 6 eggs and season them with salt and pepper to taste.

- In another pan, add the other 3 tbsps butter and let it melt over a low heat.

- Add the beaten eggs to the pan and stir for 1 minute.

- Take the sautéed vegetables and lay them over the eggs.

- Now let it sit and cook slowly for 4 minutes. Remember to not stir.

- After the omelette has set and started to brown on the bottom, fold the omelette from the side with the help of your spatula.

- Depending on how you like your omelette you can choose how long you let it set.

- Carefully remove your omelette from the pan.

TIP: For me personally, I like my omelette to be golden on the outside and creamy on the inside. So, I just let it sit for a few minutes – although this depends on the heat and power of the stove as each one is different.

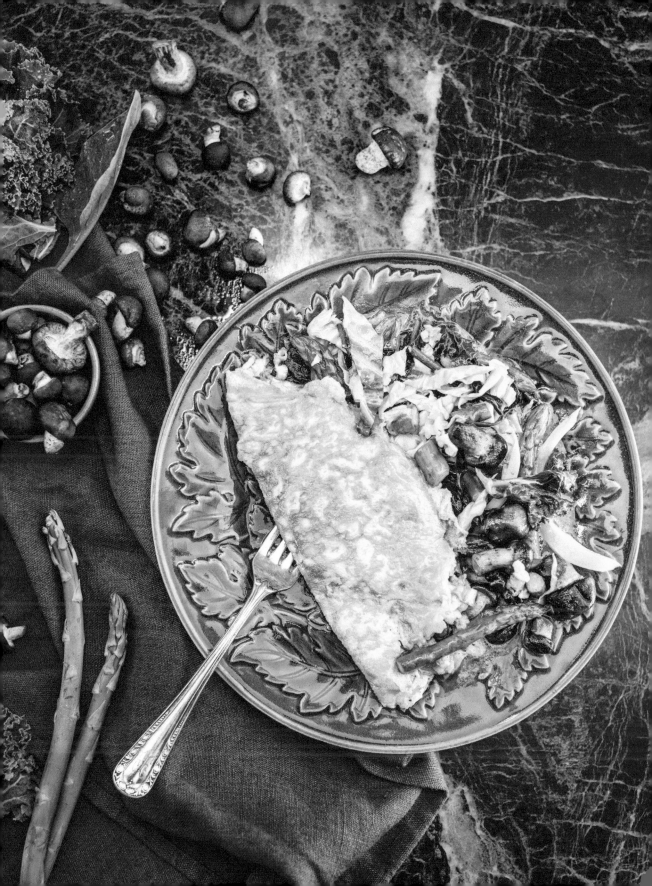

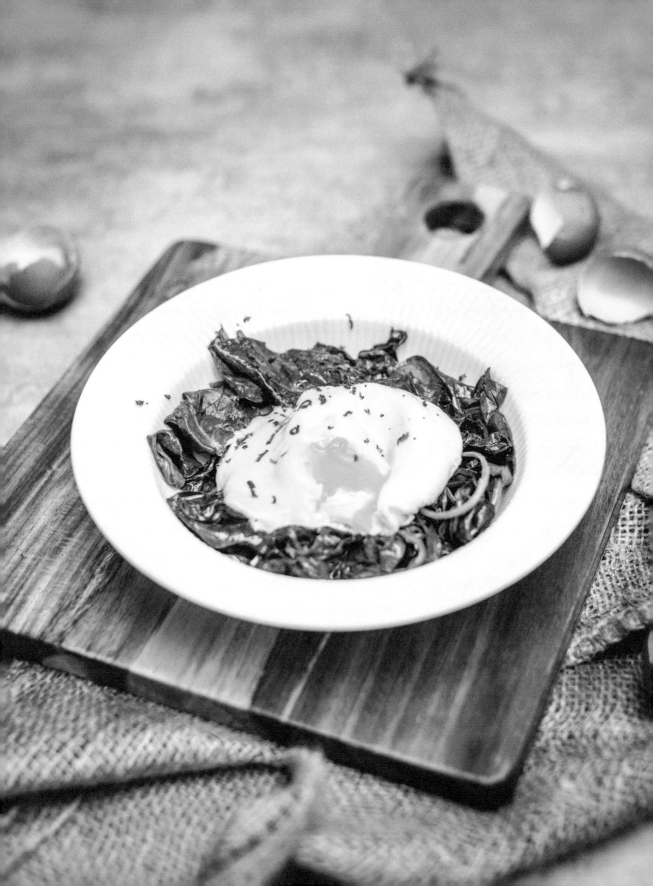

EGGS FLORENTINE WITH SPINACH AND HOLLANDAISE SAUCE

👤 Serves: **2**

⏱ Time: **30 minutes**

INGREDIENTS

300g spinach

4 eggs

fresh grated truffle

2 tbsps butter

1 tbsp apple cider vinegar or wine vinegar

salt

Hollandaise sauce
(see page 238)

UTENSILS

pan, slotted spoon

- In a pan over medium heat sauté the spinach with butter and salt for five minutes.

- Prepare the Hollandaise sauce

- Fill another frying pan with water, add a tablespoon of vinegar and put on high heat.

- After the water starts to boil, turn the heat down to medium.

- Carefully, crack the egg over the water without breaking the yolk.

- Don't stir the water or touch the egg.

- Cook each egg for 1 to 3 minutes. Cooking time will depend on how you like your egg.

- Take your slotted spoon and gently remove the egg. Make sure the water has drained and then place it on top of your cooked spinach.

- Pour the Hollandaise sauce over your egg.

- Sprinkle a little freshly grated truffle on top.

- Salt to taste.

TIP: If you have a large and deep skillet/frying pan you can make multiple eggs at once. However, if not it is best to make them one by one in order to avoid them sticking together or breaking.

AÇAI BOWL WITH KIWI, BANANA, BLUEBERRIES AND GRATED COCONUT

👤 Serves: **2**

⏱ Time: **10 minutes**

INGREDIENTS

1 tbsp açai

2 frozen bananas

64g frozen raspberries

500 ml water

32g blueberries

1 kiwi

125g strawberries

125g cashews

64g coconut flakes/grated coconut

UTENSILS

blender or food processor, knife

- Place the frozen bananas, raspberries, cashews, açai and water into the blender or food processor.

- Blend everything together until you get a nice uniform texture.

- Serve in a deep bowl.

- Wash and slice the kiwi and strawberries to your liking. Place them on top of the blended mixture in an appealing pattern and then scatter your blueberries around the bowl and finish off with some grated coconut.

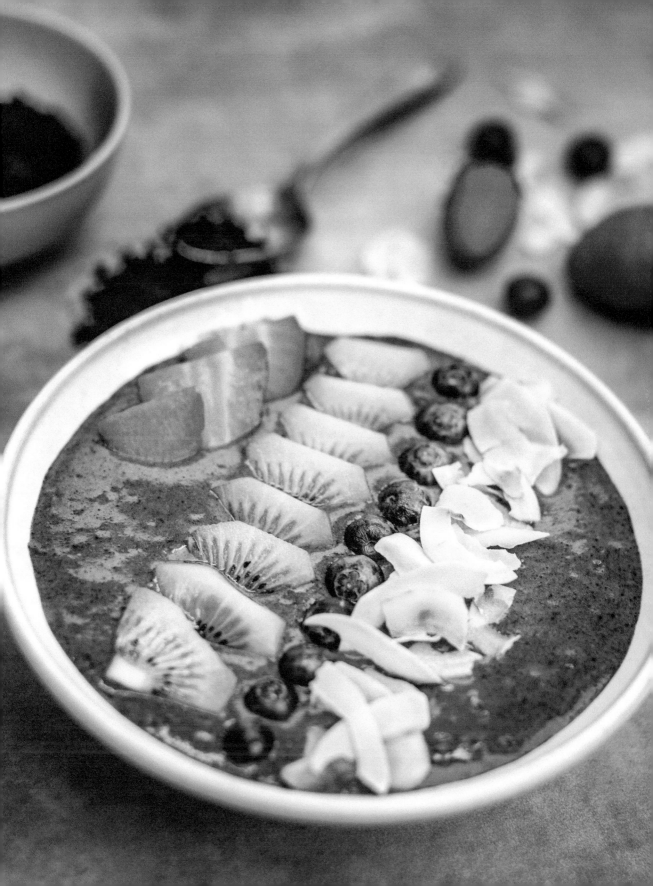

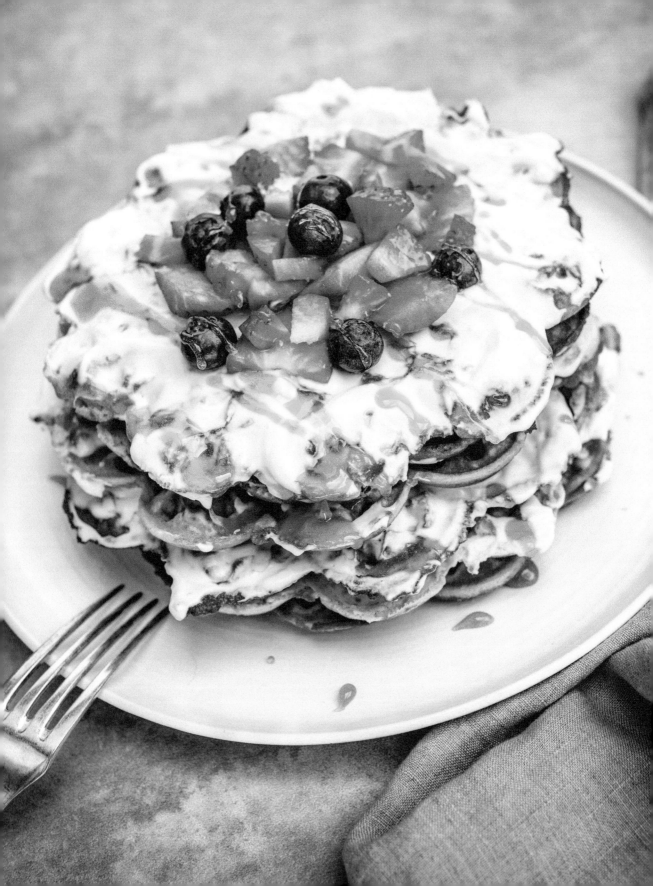

NATURAL WAFFLES

Makes: **10-12 waffles**

Time: **20 minutes**

INGREDIENTS

125g Natruly oats

125g raw cashews

64g quinoa flour

250 ml fresh whole milk

64g buckwheat flour

12 eggs

butter

UTENSILS

blender or food processor,
waffle-iron knife

- Place all your ingredients into the food processor or blender except for the milk. Blend for 5 minutes until you get a thick, uniform dough.

- Next, start to add the milk little by little, blending for 2 minutes. At this point you should turn on your waffle iron in order for it to warm up.

- Spread some butter onto each side of your waffle iron so your batter doesn't stick.

- Once hot, pour the batter into the waffle iron as you normally would. Be careful not to over-fill it so it doesn't spill over.

- Let your waffles cook for about 4-5 minutes or until your waffle iron indicates it has finished.

- When finished, remove the waffles with the help of a spatula and place them on a cooling rack.

- Now for the fun part, plating your waffles. Add any of your favourite toppings. I personally love them with yogurt, cane syrup, and fresh fruit.

TIP: Don't forget to butter your waffle iron each time you add more batter. This will not only prevent it from sticking but you will also get to enjoy its health benefits and great flavour!

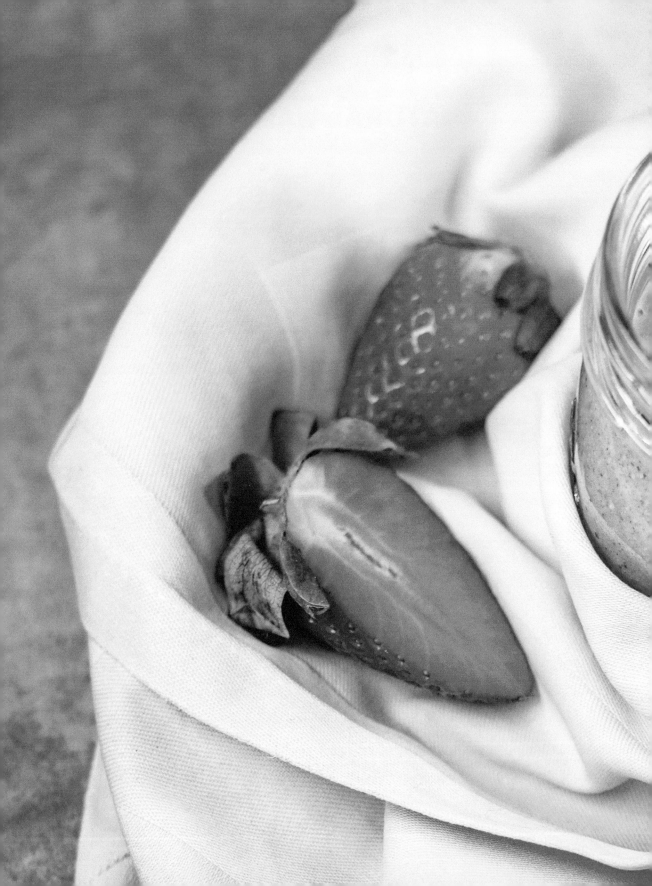

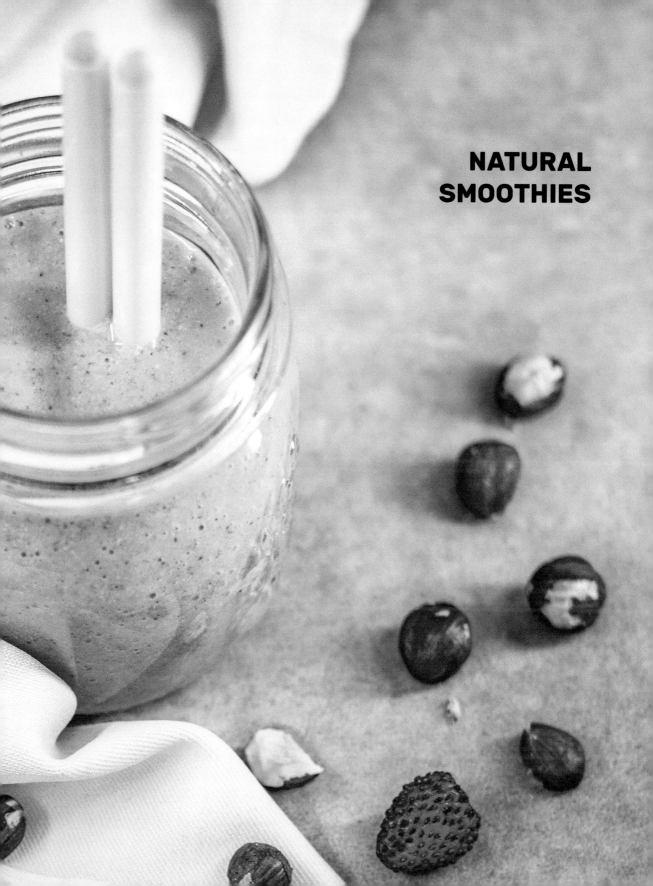

NATURAL
SMOOTHIES

BANANA AND COCOA SMOOTHIE

Serves: **2**

Time: **5-10 minutes**

INGREDIENTS

2 frozen bananas

375 ml water

42g oats

42g cashews

1 tsp cacao

1 tbsp coconut oil

UTENSILS

smoothie or food processor, knife

- The night before making, freeze two bananas that have been peeled and cut into small pieces.

- Place all the ingredients into your blender or food processor.

- Blend everything together for 5 minutes or until everything has blended together smoothly and there are no visible chunks.

- Serve your smoothie in a glass and for a nice added touch sprinkle a little cocoa and nuts on top.

TIP: You can substitute the cashews for some hazelnuts instead, it will change the flavour but, still be just as delicious!

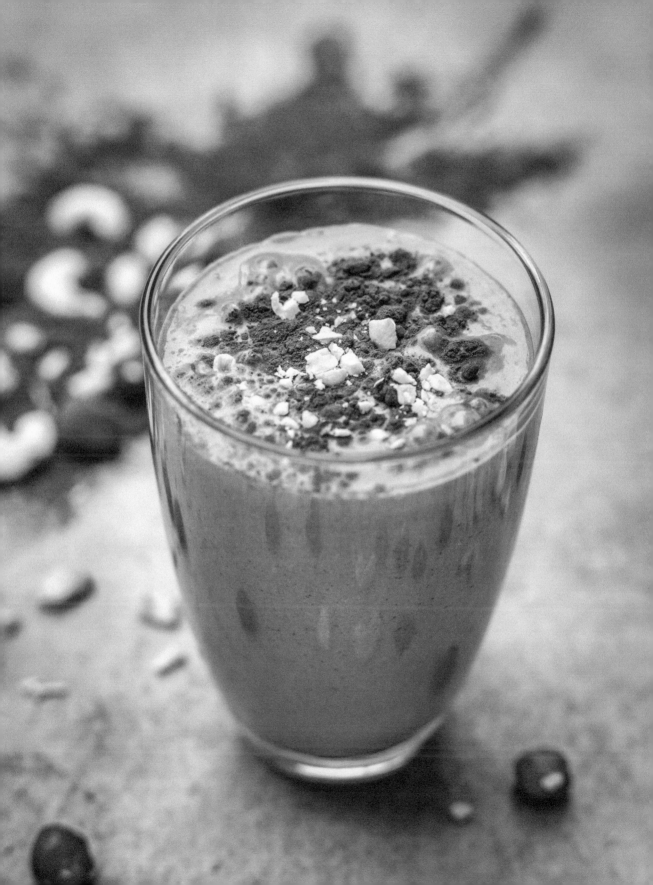

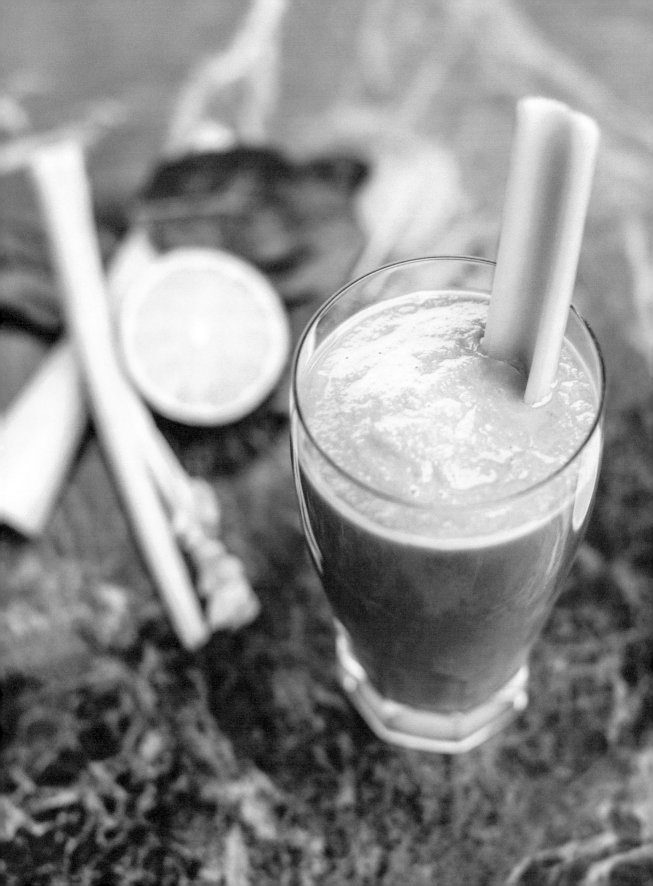

GREEN SMOOTHIE

👤 Serves: **2**

🕐 Time: **5-10 minutes**

INGREDIENTS

1 large green apple

1 small cucumber

1 avocado

handful spinach leaves

375 ml water

½ handful fresh parsley
without the stem

1 lime

1 celery stalk

1 tsp honey

1 tbsp extra virgin olive oil

pinch of salt

UTENSILS

blender or food processor,
knife, peeler

- Peel all the fruits and vegetables and extract the juice from your lime.

- Cut all peeled fruit and vegetables into smaller chunks so as not to ruin your blender.

- Wash and remove all the stems from both the spinach and the parsley.

- Place all ingredients into your blender or food processor.

- Blend for 3 minutes or until you get a uniform and creamy texture.

- Serve your smoothie in a glass and add a celery stalk for a little extra decor.

TIP: If you have a blender that is capable of crushing ice you can make this drink even more refreshing by substituting the water in the recipe with 250 ml of water and 64g ice. This will make your drink a bit cooler on those extra hot days.

WILD STRAWBERRY AND HAZELNUT SMOOTHIE

👤 Serves: **2**

⏱ Time: **5-10 minutes**

INGREDIENTS

7-9 wild strawberries

32g hazelnuts

1 frozen banana

60 ml water

UTENSILS

blender or food processor,
knife

- Make sure to freeze your banana the night before.

- Place all the ingredients into the blender and set one strawberry aside.

- Blend everything for about 5 minutes or until you have a nice uniform texture with no chunks.

- Take the strawberry that you set aside and cut it into small slices.

- Pour the smoothie mixture into your favourite glass and sprinkle the small slices of strawberry on top of the smoothie.

TIP: If you prefer your smoothie to have a creamier texture, I suggest substituting the water for whole milk instead.

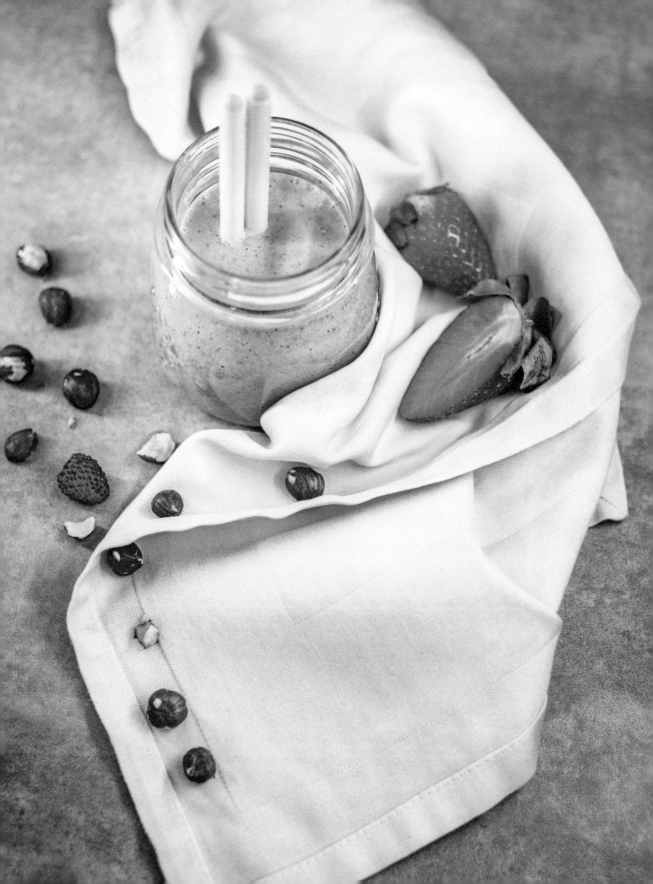

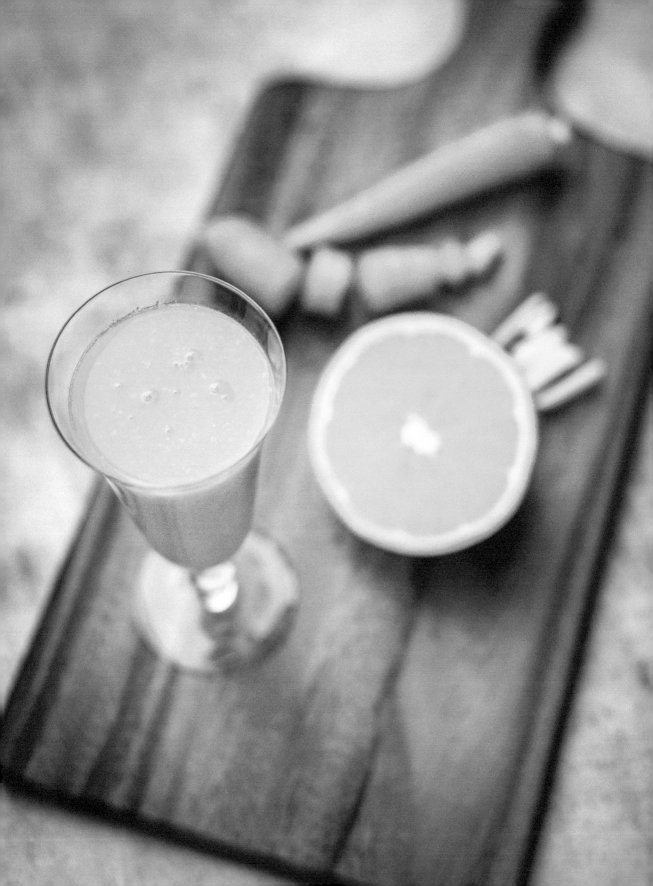

GINGER VITAMIN SMOOTHIE

👤 Serves: **2**

⏱ Time: **5-10 minutes**

INGREDIENTS

2 oranges

½ lemon

2 carrots

2 cm grated ginger

turmeric powder

250 ml water

UTENSILS

blender or food processor,
grater, juicer, peeler

- Extract the juice from your oranges and lemons using your juicer, then pour it into the blender.

- Peel the carrots and then place them in the blender as well.

- Next add the grated fresh ginger, turmeric and water.

- Blend everything for about 5 minutes or until everything has been completely blended. Make sure there are no chunks or strips of carrot left.

- Lastly pour the smoothie mixture into a glass and serve

TIP: Before you cut and juice your citrus fruit, roll them on a flat surface with the palm of your hand while applying a little pressure. This will help break up the fibres and make it easier to release its juice contents.

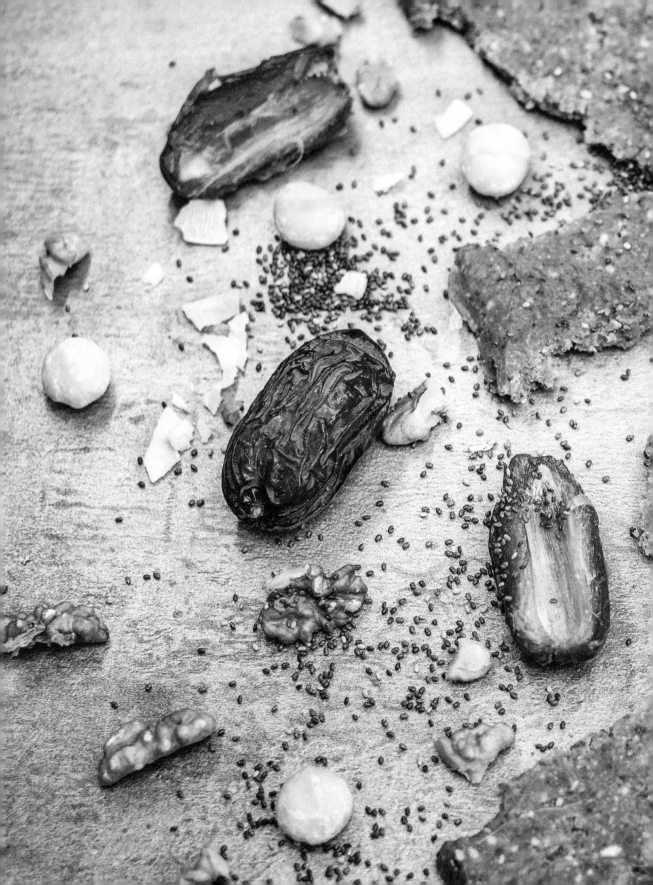

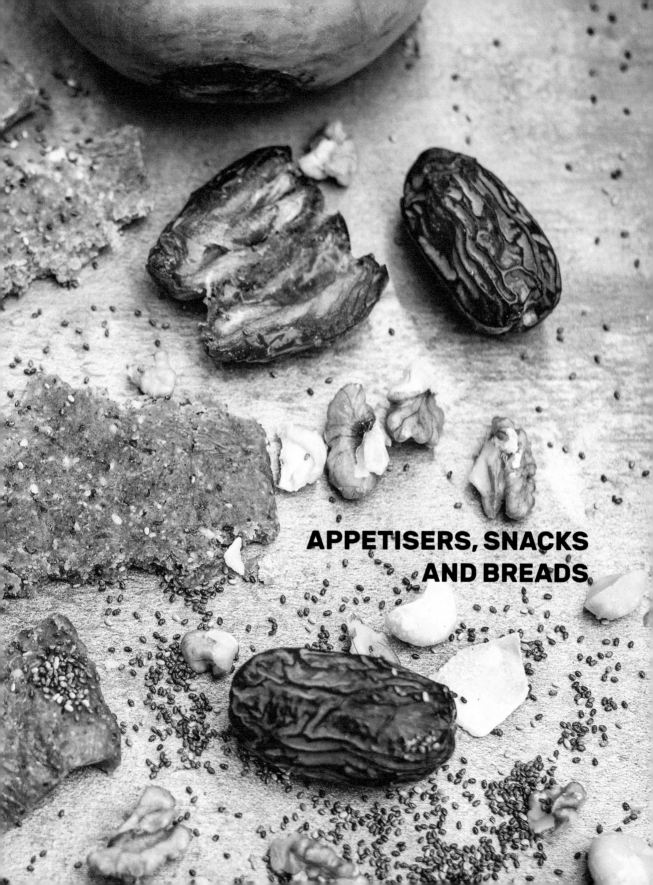

**APPETISERS, SNACKS
AND BREADS**

CRUNCHY SEED CRACKERS

👤 Serves: **4**

⏱ Time: **55 minutes**

INGREDIENTS

250 ml boiling water

32g poppy seeds

32g pumpkin seeds

32g sesame seeds

64g sunflower seeds

32g chia seeds

32g quinoa flour

32g tapioca flour

1 egg

Salt

UTENSILS

oven, oven tray, baking parchment

- Preheat the oven to 200° C.

- Take a large bowl and mix together all the different types of seeds and flour.

- Next, beat your egg in a separate small dish and then stir it into the flour and seed mixture.

- Now, start to add the boiling water little by little while you continue to stir the mixture. Do this until a dough-like texture forms.

- Add salt to taste.

- Cover the baking sheet with some wax/non-stick paper. Then pour the dough onto the baking sheet. Using your hands, spread the dough until the entire surface of the baking sheet is covered with a thin layer. Make sure that it is evenly spread out.

- Place the baking sheet into the pre-heated oven and bake for 45 minutes.

- Remove it from the oven when it starts to get a nice golden colour. Let it sit and cool.

- Break off pieces from the bread using your hands. These gluten-free crackers are great for making canapes.

TIP: If you prefer to have each cracker the same size – before placing the dough into the oven, take a knife and cut the dough into your preferred shape and size.

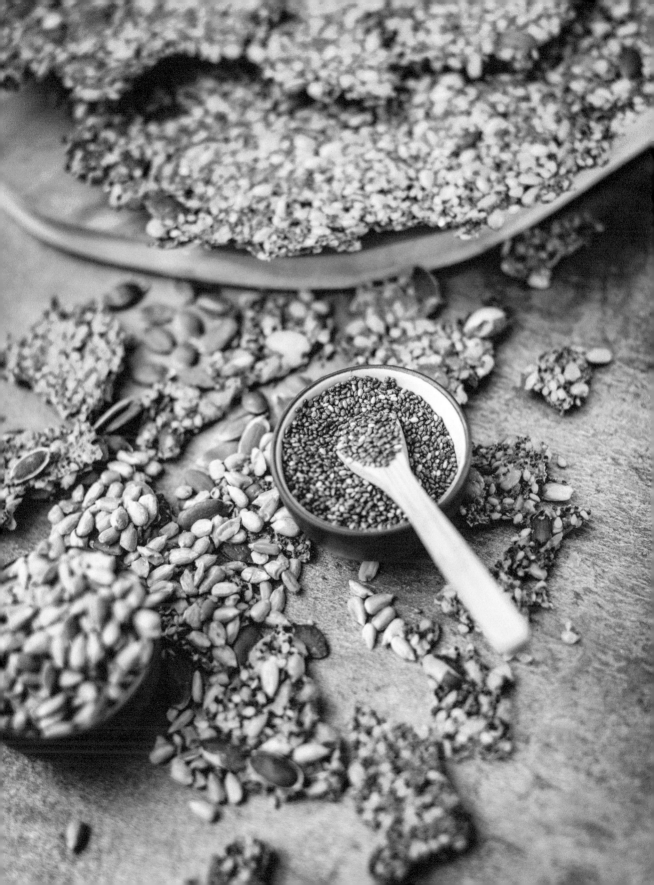

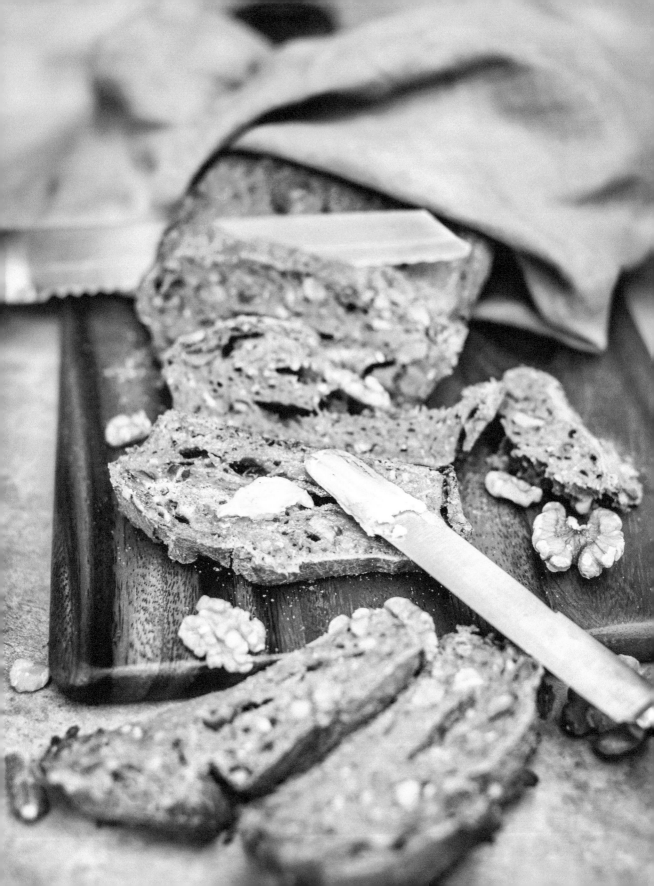

CHIA AND WALNUT BREAD

👤 Serves: **4**

⏱ Time: **10 minutes + 1 hour**

INGREDIENTS

5 eggs

125g tapioca flour

64g buckwheat flour

64g peeled walnuts

64g chia flour

2 tbsps butter

3 tbsps extra virgin olive oil

chia seeds

UTENSILS

oven, loaf/cake tin, baking parchment, spatula, whisk

- Preheat oven to 180° C.

- Mix all the flours together in a big bowl.

- Add salt to taste.

- Crack each egg one by one over the dry ingredients. Stir each egg with the whisk, integrating it into the flour before cracking the next egg. That way you will get a better and more uniform dough.

- Before adding the last egg, add the olive oil and room-temperature butter.

- Lastly, add the chia seeds and walnuts. Combine well.

- Grease the loaf/cake tin with some butter or cover it with some non-stick paper.

- Fill the loaf/cake tin with the dough and bake for 1 hour.

- Remove it from the oven when it is has cooked and turned a golden-brown color. Let it rest for a few minutes after removing it from the oven. This bread is ideal for making sandwiches and canapes.

TIP: If you have a mixer with blades capable of making bread dough, you can use that and save time. Keep in mind that the consistency of this dough won't be quite the same as regular bread dough.

DATE, NUTS AND CHIA BARS

Makes: **12-16** bars

Time: **10 minutes + 2 hours**

INGREDIENTS

500g dates (25 pieces)

125g natural cashews

125g natural or roasted almonds with skin

125g toasted hazelnuts

32g chia

64g coconut flour

100 ml coconut oil

1 tsp salt

UTENSILS

Food Processor, baking tray, non-stick paper/baking parchment, pizza cutter or thin knife

- Grind separately the cashews, hazelnuts and almonds in a food processor. Each nut should turn into a flour-like powder.

- Mix all the nut-flours and chia together in a large bowl and set aside.

- Remove the stones from the dates and then grind the dates in the food processor until they form a paste. Pour that paste into the large bowl.

- Add the coconut flour, salt and coconut oil. Stir everything together until a uniform dough is formed.

- Cover the baking tray with a sheet of non-stick paper. Then place the dough on the tray and flatten it out with your hands or by using a rolling pin. Stretch the dough into a flat rectangle that is about half a centimetre thick.

- Cut the dough into rectangular squares using the pizza cutter. They can be any size you want.

- Place the tray into the freezer for at least 2 hours.

- Keep the bars stored in an airtight container in the refrigerator. You can store your gluten-free bars in the freezer for months.

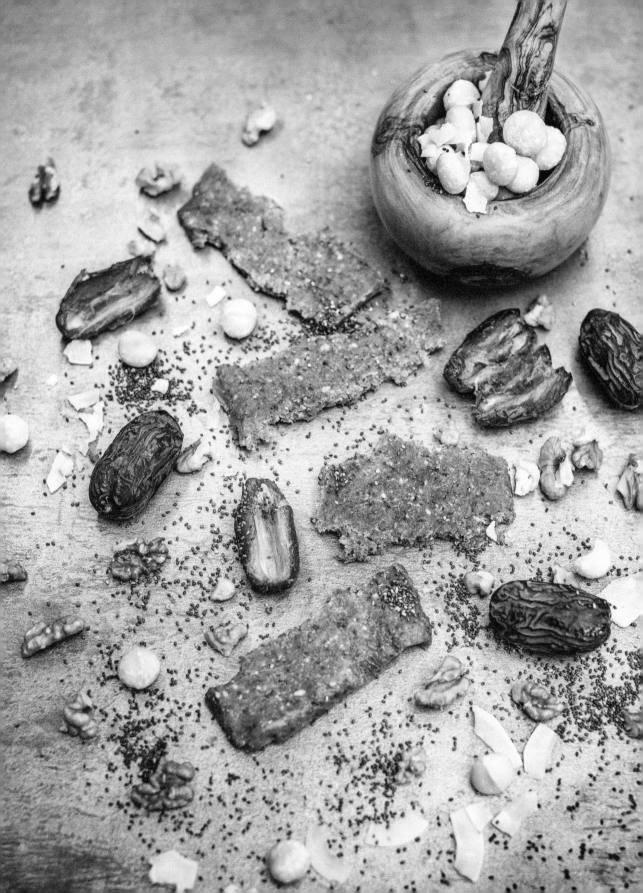

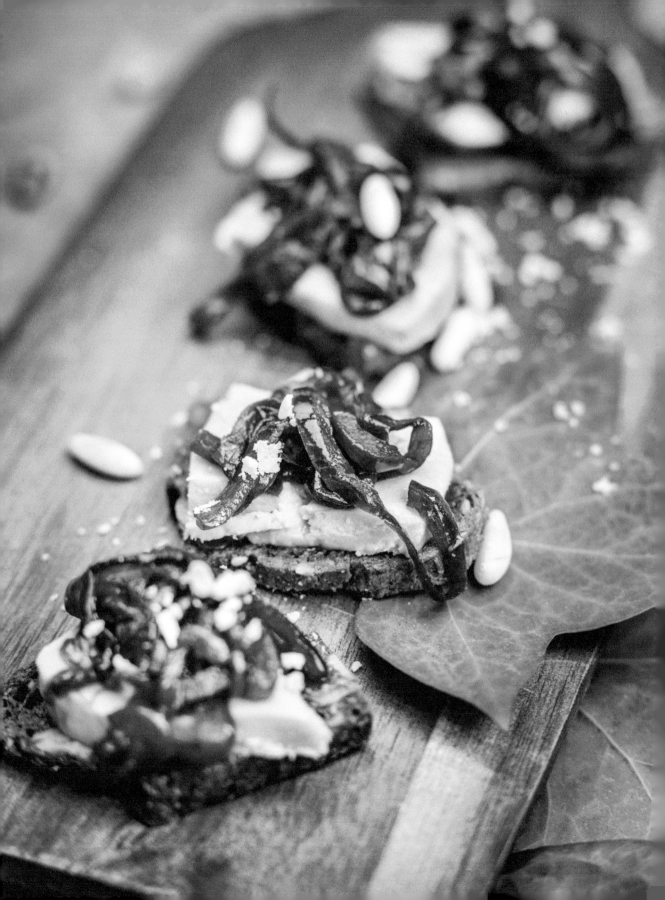

FOIE GRAS CANAPES WITH CARAMELISED ONION

Serves: **4**

Time: **30 minutes**

INGREDIENTS

250g organic foie gras

4 red onions

8 slices bread

butter

salt

UTENSILS

frying pan, knife without serrated edges

- Cut the onion into strips.

- In a frying pan over medium heat, add a slice of butter and let it start to melt. Next add your onions.

- Add some salt to taste and let the onions begin to sweat.

- Don't stir the onions until they start to turn a golden colour.

- Lower the heat and let the onion caramelise for about 20 minutes, stirring them from time to time.

- Take the sliced bread and split them into smaller pieces. The canapes should be bite sized.

- In a clean frying pan with a little butter, brown each slice of bread on both sides.

- The foie gras should be at room temperature. When it is, slice it into small pieces using a thin, sharp knife without serrated edges.

- Place a piece of foie gras on each canapé and top it with some caramelised onion.

TIP: In order to cut the foie gras in a way so that it doesn't stick or break, you should soak your knife in hot water and then dry it well before cutting each piece of foie gras. Always clean the knife between cuts so you can ensure the perfect slice each and every time.

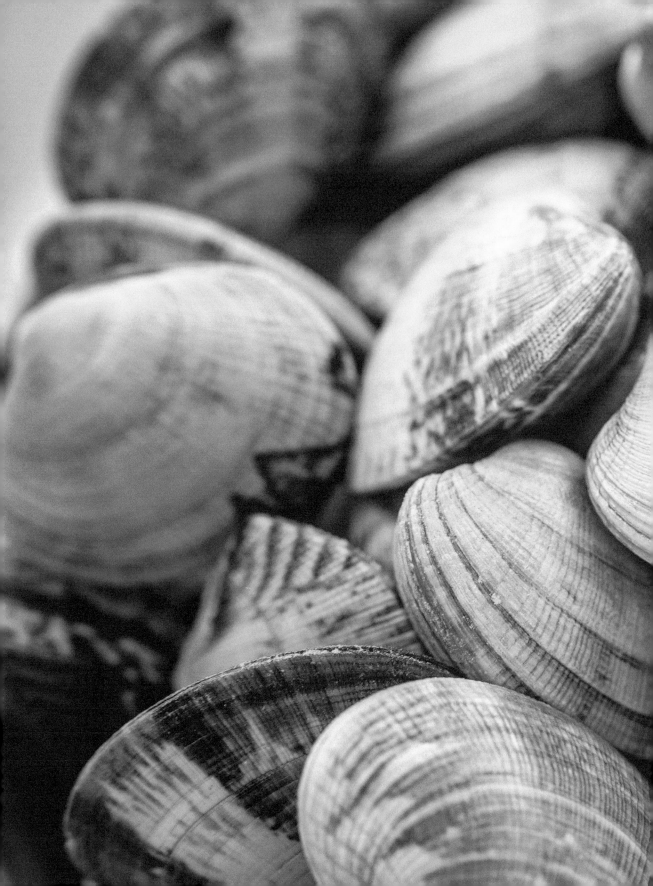

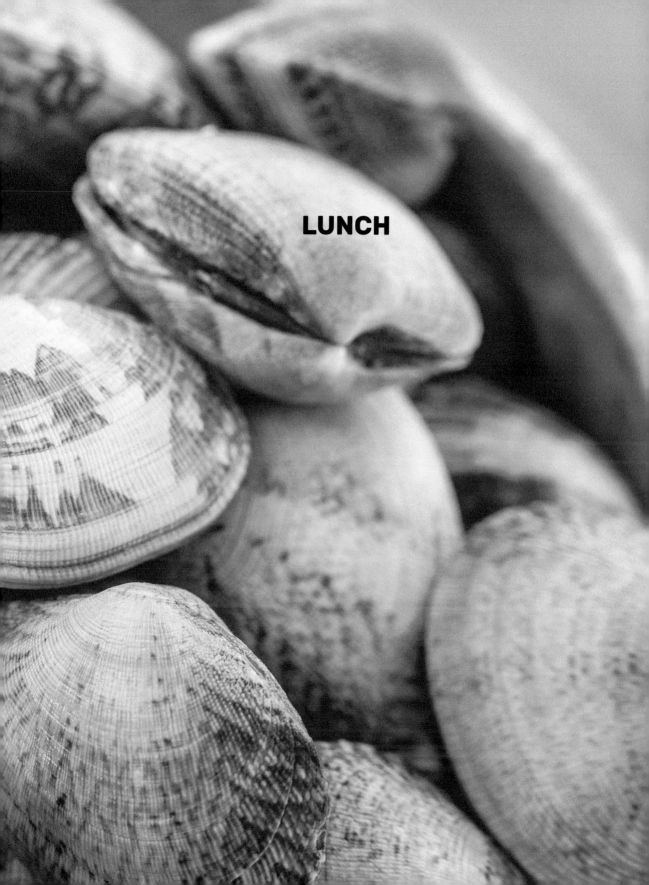

LUNCH

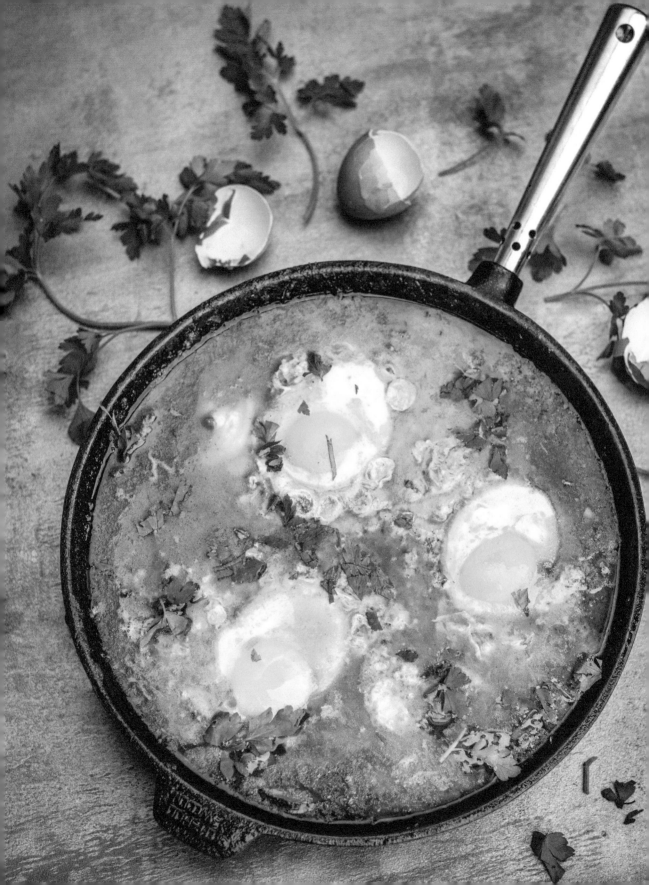

SHAKSHUKA

Serves: **3**

Time: **30 minutes**

INGREDIENTS

2 courgettes

2 mozzarella balls

3 eggs

1 red pepper

fresh parsley

butter

salt

500g tomato sauce
(see page 239)

UTENSILS

large pan, knife

- Slice the courgettes and dice the red pepper into pieces and then cook it in butter for 10 minutes over medium heat.

- Add the tomato sauce (see page 239) and mix it in well.

- Slice the mozzarella into thin slices and spread them out on top of the sauce throughout the pan.

- Using a spoon, make three holes in the sauce where the eggs can be placed.

- When the sauce is bubbling, carefully crack an egg into each hollowed out place.

- Cook the eggs over medium-low heat. Once the whites of the eggs have turned white, remove the shakshuka from the heat and garnish with some chopped parsley.

TIP: If you don't want to risk it, crack the eggs in a separate bowl and then pour them into the sauce one by one. That way you don't have to worry about any yolks breaking and you can get the perfect dish.

ROASTED AUBERGINE SALAD WITH GOAT'S CHEESE

👤 Serves: **2-4**

⏱ Time: **20 minutes**

INGREDIENTS

2 aubergines

200g goat's cheese

toasted pine nuts to taste

1 pomegranate

salt and pepper

extra virgin olive oil

4-5 fresh basil leaves

UTENSILS

skillet or pan, paper towel, knife

- Cut the aubergines into half centimetre slices.

- Add salt to each slice on both sides. Let it sit and then dry off each slice with a paper towel, soaking up all the water.

- Drizzle some olive oil into your pan. Cook the aubergine over medium heat until both sides are golden brown.

- Remove from heat and drain any excess oil.

- Cut the cheese into small pieces and remove the seeds from the pomegranate.

- Sprinkle the cheese over the aubergine slices along with the pine nuts and pomegranate seeds.

- Serve this in a bowl and decorate with some added basil leaves.

TIP: To remove the seeds from the pomegranate, just cut it in half horizontally and use your hands to carefully open it. Then face the cut side down, and gently tap it with a spoon until the seeds start to fall out. Do this until all of them have been removed.

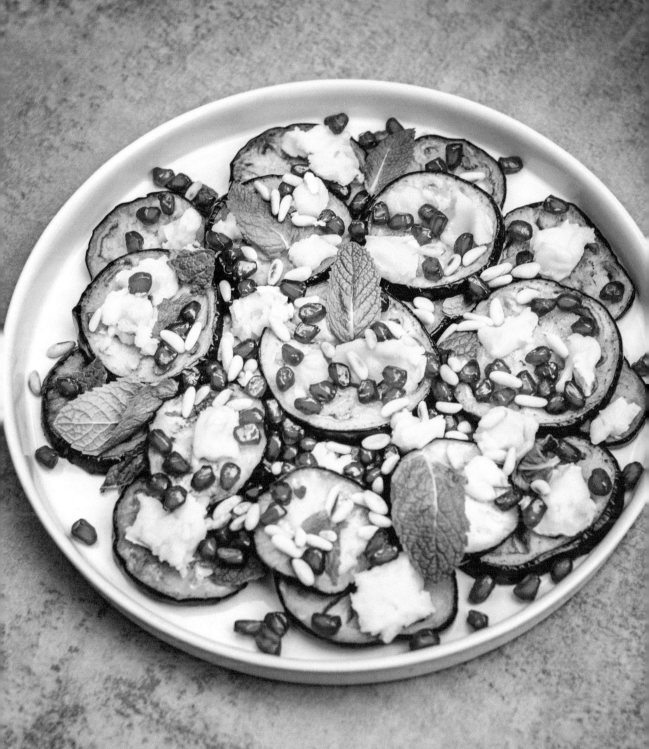

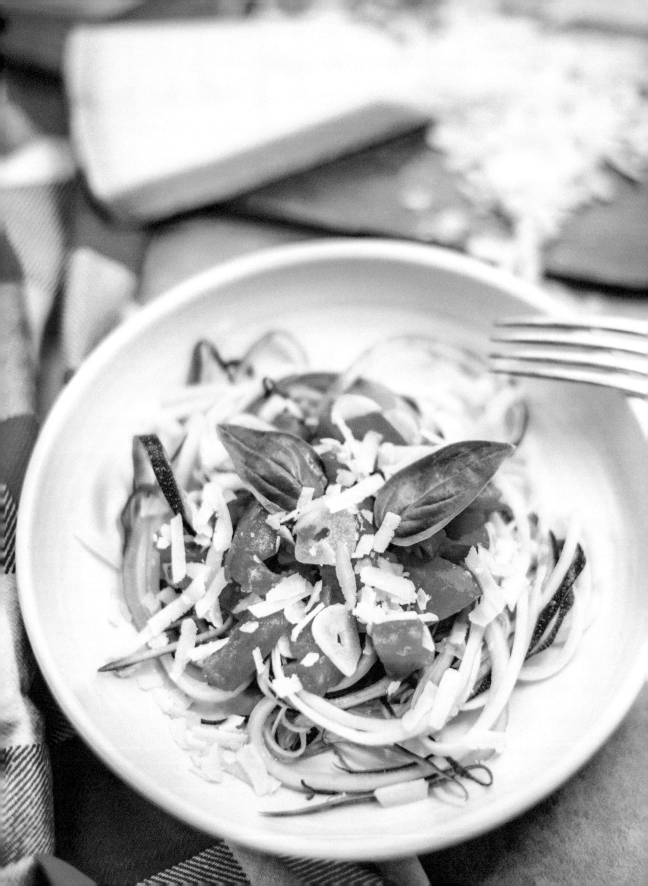

COURGETTI WITH TOMATOES AND BASIL

👤 Serves: **2**

🕐 Time: **20 minutes**

INGREDIENTS

1 large courgette

4 tomatoes

1 clove garlic

salt and pepper

1 tbsp butter

extra virgin olive oil

parmesan cheese

32g fresh basil

UTENSILS

spiraliser, grater (optional)

- Chop the tomatoes and garlic into small pieces.

- Melt the butter in the frying pan and sauté the tomato and garlic for 4-5 minutes. Salt and pepper to taste.

- Rinse your courgette well. Using the spiraliser, cut into thin noodle-like strips.

- Boil the courgetti for 1-2 minutes until they are al dente.

- Strain the courgetti. Then place a serving of the courgetti on a plate and top them with the sautéed tomatoes and garlic.

- Grate some parmesan cheese over the courgetti. You can also cut the parmesan into thin slices if you prefer. Add as much or as little as you like.

- For the final touch, drizzle some extra virgin olive oil on top and place some fresh basil leaves all over the dish.

TIP: There are many spiralisers to choose from and any of them will work for this recipe or for any recipe where you want to make noodles out of vegetables.

KALE AND SPINACH CREAM SOUP WITH PARMESAN CRISPS

Serves: **2**

Time: **20 minutes**

INGREDIENTS

200g kale

200g spinach

150g parmesan

50g natural mayonnaise
(see page 240)

100 ml fresh cream

1 litre broth or water
(see page 193)

salt

4 tbsps butter

poppy seeds

UTENSILS

oven, blender or food
processor, knife

- Preheat oven to 225° C.

- Cut the parmesan into wide strips. They don't have to be the same size.

- Place the parmesan onto a baking sheet and sprinkle each piece with a few poppy seeds. Bake for 10 minutes or until each strip is golden brown and crispy.

- Fill a pot with the broth of your choice and cook the spinach and kale together over medium heat. Using bone broth is a great option for this recipe – however, if you don't have any broth on hand, use the same amount of water and just add a little salt to taste.

- Once the vegetables are tender, remove them from the heat and let sit for 5-10 minutes.

- Next, blend the vegetables together in a food processor or blender creating a smooth and creamy soup texture.

- Mix the mayonnaise and fresh cream together in a separate bowl.

- Pour the cream soup into a bowl and decorate the top by drizzling some of the mayo-cream sauce in a circular motion. Place a parmesan chip or two on the side and enjoy!

TIP: If you want your cream soup to be even smoother, strain it through a fine mesh strainer.

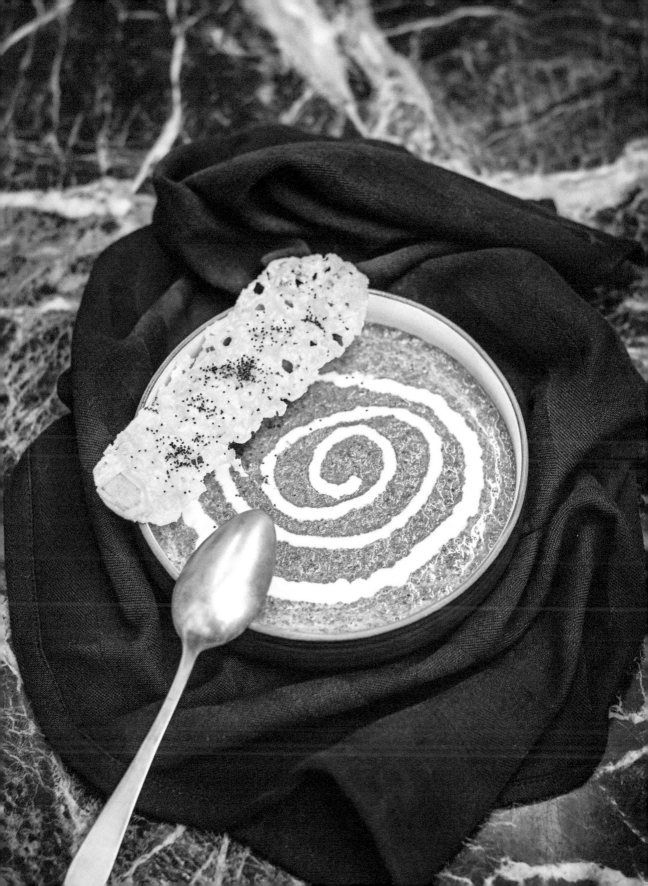

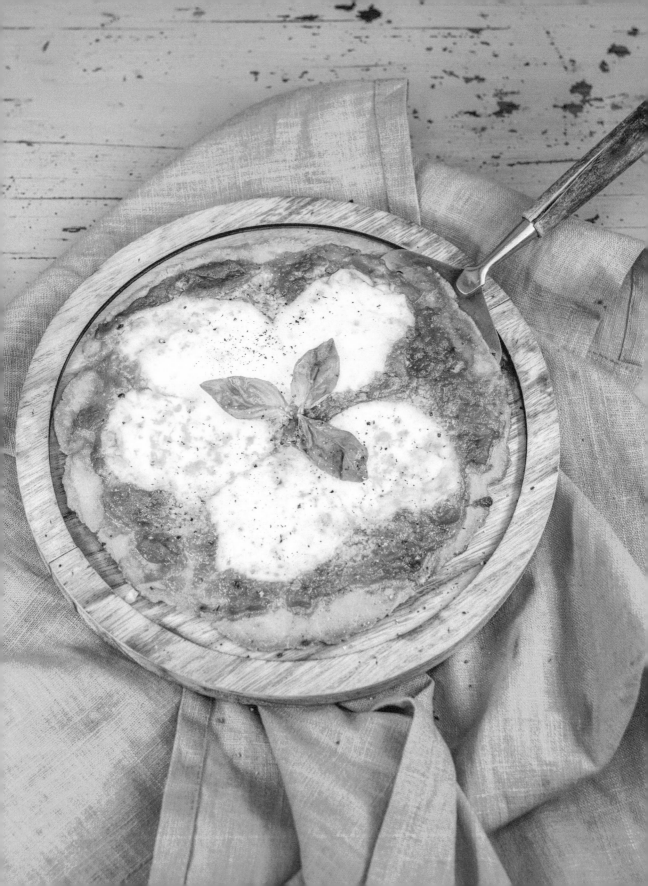

NAPOLITANA PIZZA

👤 Serves: **1**

🕓 Time: **20 minutes**

INGREDIENTS

pizza base

125g almond flour

125g coconut flour

1 large egg

salt

olive oil (optional)

pizza topping

64g tomato sauce
(see page 239)

1 mozzarella ball

black pepper

4-6 basil leaves

UTENSILS

oven, baking parchment,
baking tray

- Preheat oven to 175 ºC.

- Prepare the dough for the base of the pizza:

- Mix all the ingredients for the dough together in one bowl.

- You want the dough to be firm so adjust the quantities as needed. If the dough is too runny add more almond flour. If the dough is too thick drizzle in some more olive oil.

- Stretch the dough out with your hands making a circular shape and then place it onto the baking tray.

- Prepare the pizza toppings:

- Spread the tomato sauce on top of the pizza dough using a spoon and bake it in the oven for 10 minutes.

- Remove the pizza and place the sliced mozzarella on top of the pizza along with the fresh basil leaves and black pepper.

- Place it back in the oven and bake for another 5 minutes.

TIP: For more flavour, add some bacon, chopped onions or capers to the pizza.

CRÉME FRAÎCHE PIZZA WITH SALMON EGGS AND RED ONION

👤 Serves: **1**

⏱ Time: **20 minutes**

INGREDIENTS

pizza base

125g almond flour

125g coconut flour

1 large egg

salt

olive oil (optional)

pizza topping

100 parmesan

½ red onion

1 tbsp sour cream

32g chives

2 tbsps salmon eggs

UTENSILS

oven, baking parchment, knife, baking tray, grater

- Preheat oven to 175° C.

- Prepare dough for pizza base:

- Mix all the ingredients for the dough together in one bowl.

- You want the dough to be firm so adjust the quantities as needed. If the dough is too runny add more almond flour. If the dough is too thick drizzle in some more olive oil.

- Stretch the dough out with your hands making a circular shape and then place it onto the baking tray.

- Prepare pizza toppings:

- Grate the parmesan cheese.

- Sprinkle the grated cheese on top of the pizza dough. Place it in the oven and bake for 12 minutes.

- Remove from the oven and let cool for a few minutes. While the pizza is cooling, dice the onion and chives.

- Once the pizza has cooled, place all the ingredients on top of the pizza and serve.

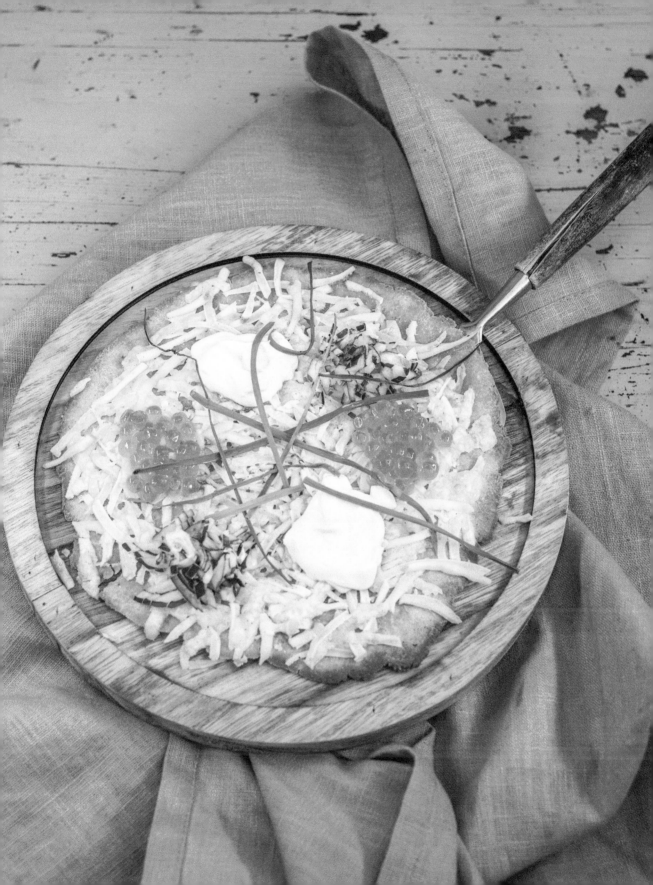

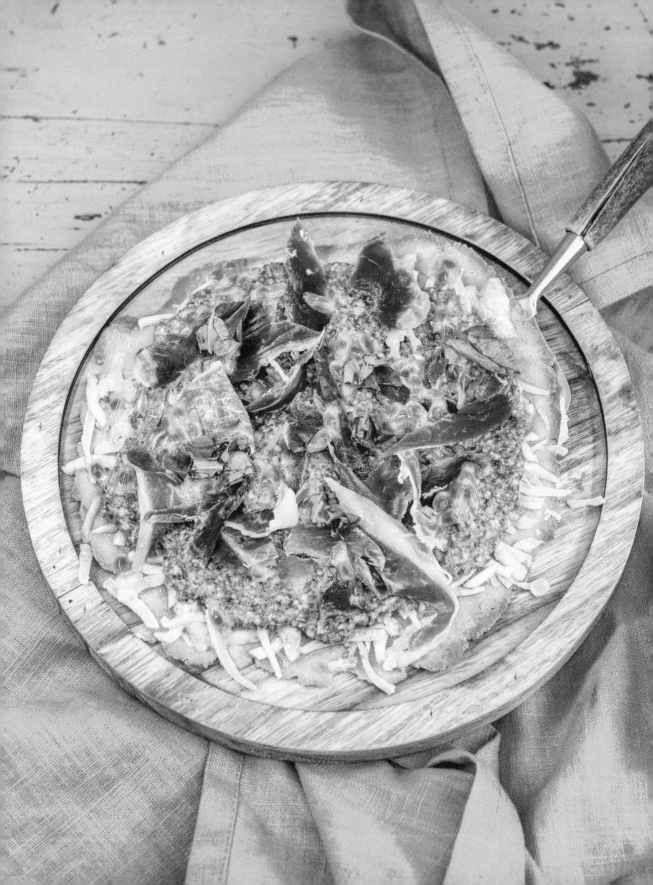

PASSION FRUIT AND IBERIAN HAM PIZZA

Serves: **1**

Time: **20 minutes**

INGREDIENTS

pizza base

125g almond flour

125g coconut flour

1 large egg

salt

olive oil (optional)

pizza topping

100g parmesan

3 tbsps pesto (see page 220)

2 tbsps passion fruit

80g acorn-fed Iberian ham

4-6 basil leaves

UTENSILS

oven, baking parchment,
baking tray, knife, grater

- Preheat oven to 175° C.

- Prepare dough for pizza base:

- Mix all the ingredients for the dough together in one bowl.

- You want the dough to be firm so adjust the quantities as needed. If the dough is too runny add more almond flour. If the dough is too thick drizzle in some more olive oil.

- Stretch the dough out with your hands making a circular shape and then place it onto the baking tray.

- Prepare the pizza toppings:

- Grate the parmesan cheese.

- Sprinkle the grated cheese on top of the pizza dough. Place it in the oven and bake for 12 minutes.

- Remove the pizza from the oven and let cool for a few minutes. While it cools dice up your Iberian ham into small pieces.

- Spread the pesto sauce over the cheese.

- Lastly, place all the toppings onto the pizza and enjoy!

TIP: Drizzle some extra virgin olive oil on top for an even juicier pizza.

ROASTED PINEAPPLE WITH TUNA BELLY

Serves: **2**

Time: **10 minutes**

INGREDIENTS

1 pineapple

400g tuna belly

32g chives

UTENSILS

large knife, grill

- Using a large knife, cut the pineapple in half. Grill each half on the side with the skin. Let it grill for 8 minutes over medium heat.

- Flip the pineapple over and let it cook for another 8 minutes.

- Remove it from the grill and place the tuna belly in the centre of the pineapple.

- Dice some chives and sprinkle it all over your pineapple and it's ready!

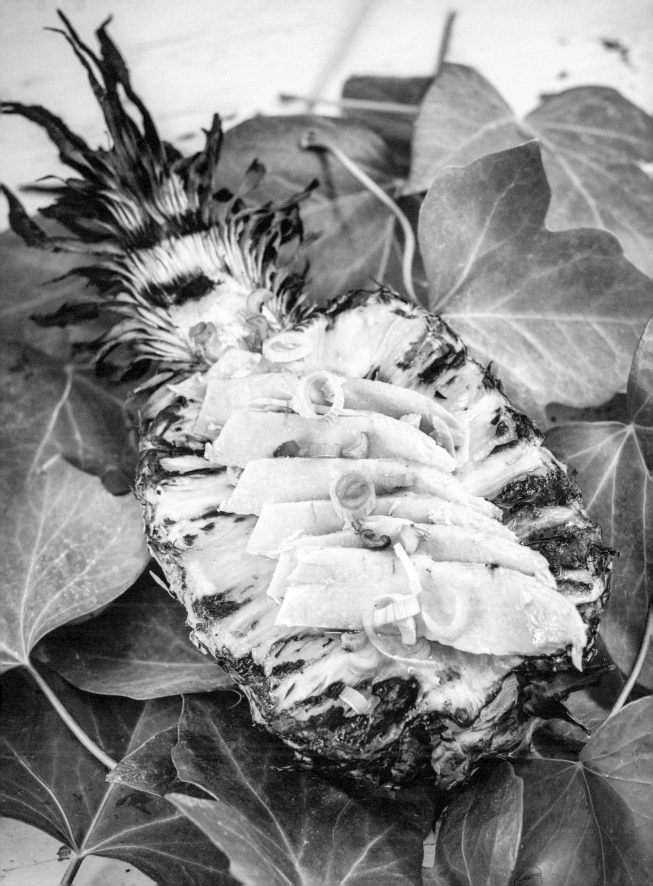

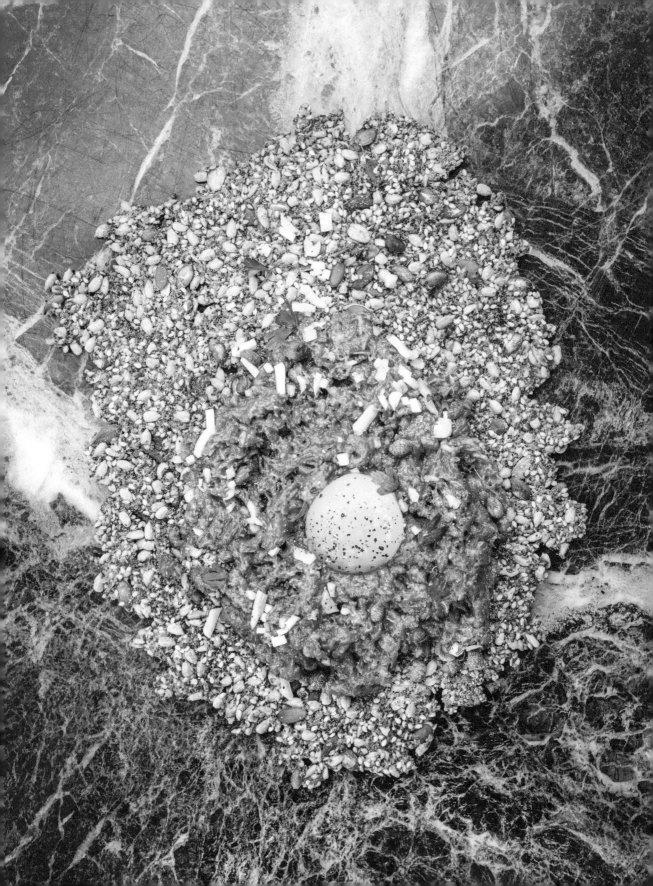

VENISON TARTARE WITH SEEDED CRIPSBREAD

👤 Serves: **2**

⏱ Time: **10 minutes**

INGREDIENTS

300g venison

2 tbsps extra virgin olive oil

1 tbsp Dijon mustard

1 egg yolk

salt

black pepper

capers

1 onion

parsley

hot sauce

crispbread (see page 158)

UTENSILS

very sharp meat cleaver

- Mince the meat with the help of a very sharp meat cleaver until you get a smooth and uniform texture.

- Mix the meat with the oil, mustard and a few drops of hot sauce. Season to taste with salt and pepper.

- Use a piece of crispbread as a base.

- Take a spoon and spread out some of the meat mixture onto the crispbread. Form a circle that is about 1½ cm thick.

- Next, make an indentation on top of the meat using the spoon. This is where you will place the egg yolk.

- Crack the egg and separate the egg whites from the egg yolk. Be sure not to break the yolk.

- Place the egg yolk in the indentation that you previously made in the meat.

- Top the dish with chopped onion, capers and parsley.

TIP: If you want your dish to look like it was plated at a restaurant, use a round mould or ring to plate the tartare meat mixture. This will give you the perfect circular shape.

MINI HAMBURGERS

👤 Serves: **2**

⏱ Time: **25 minutes**

INGREDIENTS

300g ground beef

2 egg yolks

1 avocado

1 tomato

½ onion

4 lettuce leaves

1 ball mozzarella cheese

250 ml homemade
mayonnaise (see page 240)

250 ml barbecue sauce
(see page 241)

2 tbsps butter

salt and pepper

UTENSILS

pan or grill, knife

- Mix the ground beef with the two egg yolks and season to taste.

- Split the ground beef into individual pieces that weigh about 150g each.

- Using your hands, form a ball with the ground beef and press down slightly shaping the patty to your liking.

- Grill the patty for about 3-6 minutes on each side, depending on how you like your meat.

- Meanwhile, cut all the vegetables and the mozzarella cheese into slices.

- Mix together the homemade mayo and barbecue sauce, creating a rose-coloured dressing.

- Assemble the hamburger by using the lettuce as a base and then placing all the ingredients you like on top.

TIP: If you prefer the cheese to be melted on top, just remember to place it on the burger when you flip it over to grill on the other side.

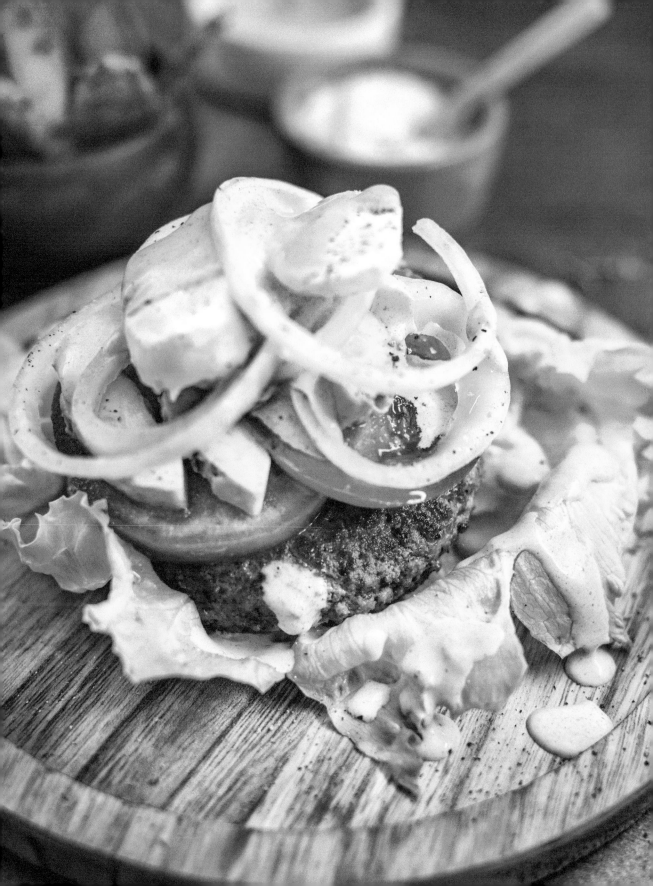

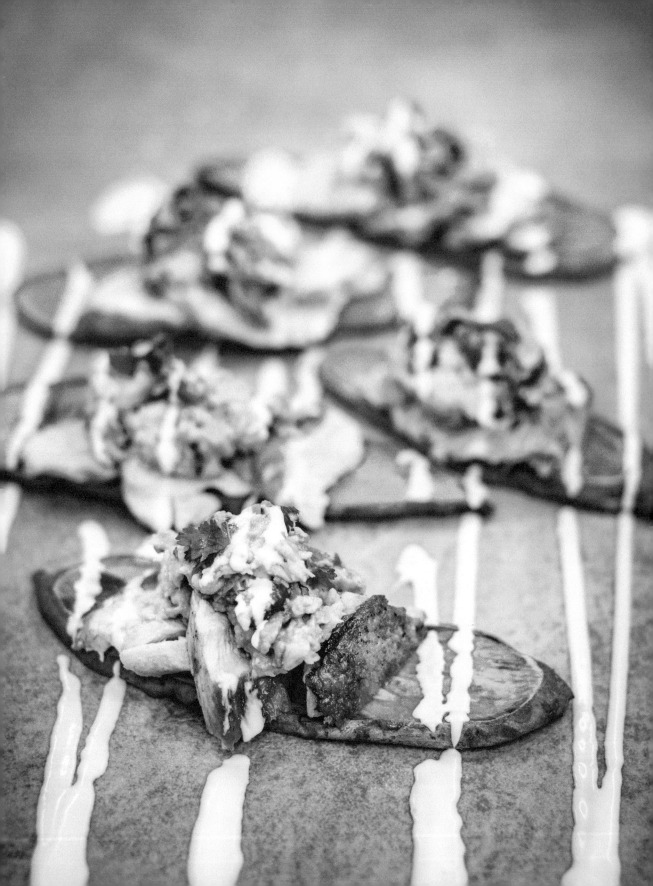

CHICKEN WITH SWEET POTATO FAJITAS

Serves: **2**

Time: **50 minutes**

INGREDIENTS

2 sweet potatoes

2 tbsps avocado oil

1 large chicken breast with the skin or 2 small chicken breasts.

100g homemade guacamole (see page 242)

60 ml thick dairy cream

60 ml natural, homemade mayo (see page 240)

salt and pepper

UTENSILS

pan, oven, knife

- Preheat oven to 180° C.

- With the skin still on, slice the sweet potatoes into long pieces that are ½ cm thick.

- Season them to taste and drizzle some avocado oil over the slices.

- Place the slices on a baking sheet and bake for 20 minutes; remove from oven and flip the slices over and bake another 20 minutes.

- Pour a tablespoon of avocado oil in a pan.

- Season the chicken breast on both sides. Place it in the pan and let cook. The chicken will release fat; leave it until browned and then flip it over and cook on the other side.

- In a bowl, mix together the homemade natural mayonnaise with the thick cream and set aside.

- Remove the sweet potatoes from the oven.

- After the chicken has cooked, remove it from the pan and cut it into strips.

- Assemble the fajita by placing the chicken strips and the guacamole on top of the baked sweet potato strips. Drizzle with some of the white sauce mixture and garnish with chopped parsley.

TIP: If you decide to make your chicken or guacamole spicy, keep the white sauce in the refrigerator and serve it cold. This will offset the spiciness and add a lot of freshness to the dish.

MOUSSAKA WITH TZATZIKI

Serves: **4**

Time: **2 hours**

INGREDIENTS

1 onion

4 garlic cloves

500g lamb (mutton)

500g aubergine

250 ml extra virgin olive oil

2 tomatoes

1 tsp cinnamon powder

2-3 fresh mint leaves

50g freshly chopped parsley

50 ml white wine

200g grated semi-cured cheese

250 ml tapioca bechamel sauce (see page 244)

tzatziki sauce (see page 243)

UTENSILS

pan, absorbent paper towel, large pot, baking dish, knife

- Preheat oven to 180° C.

- Slice the aubergine into ½ cm thick pieces. Sprinkle salt on top of the slices and let sit for 30 minutes. This will release the water from the aubergine slices.

- Wash the aubergine with cold water and dry with some extra absorbent paper towels.

- Pour some olive oil in a pan and fry the aubergine slices.

- After they turn a golden brown colour remove them from the pan and place them on some paper towel to remove the excess oil.

- Blanch the tomatoes, then peel and cut into pieces.

- Dice up the onion and garlic. Mince the lamb and add salt and pepper to taste.

- In a large pot, add 3 tbsps olive oil and sauté the onion and garlic. Next, add the minced meat and sauté over medium-low heat.

- Add the mint, parsley and cinnamon. Cook for 10 minutes. Now add the tomatoes and a splash of white wine and let it cook until the liquid is reduced and you get a thick sauce.

- Grease the baking dish with a little olive oil. Cover the bottom of the dish with a layer of aubergine slices. Then spread a layer of the meat on top. Repeat this process.

- On the last layer, pour the tapioca bechamel over the top and sprinkle some grated cheese on top.

- Place in the oven and bake for 25 minutes and another 5 minutes with the oven set high, to brown.

- Let the moussaka rest for 5 minutes before serving. Serve with tzatziki sauce or yogurt and garnish with fresh parsley.

TIP: I wanted to make this dish as an appetiser so, I did the same process but just with an individual slice of aubergine instead of layering.

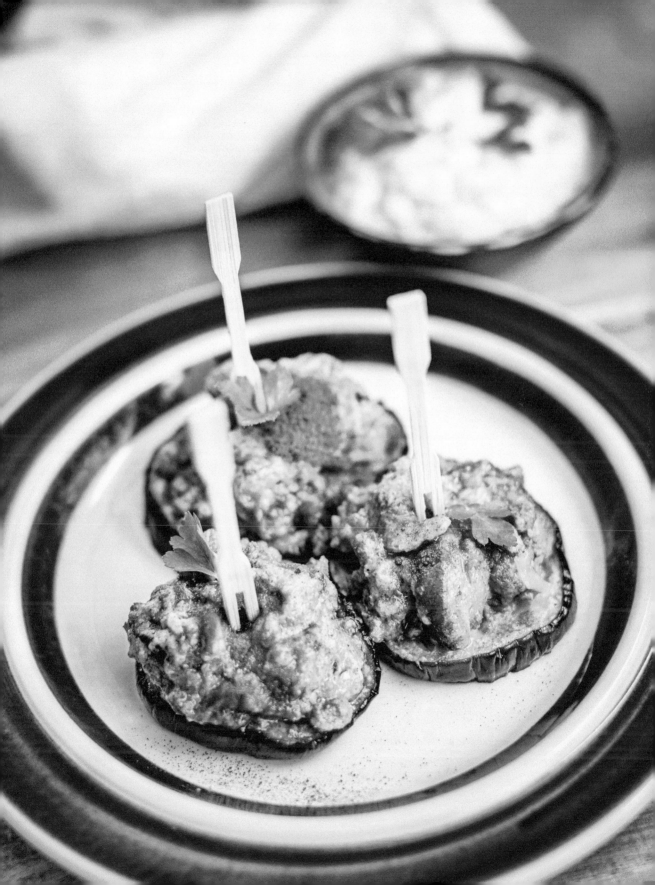

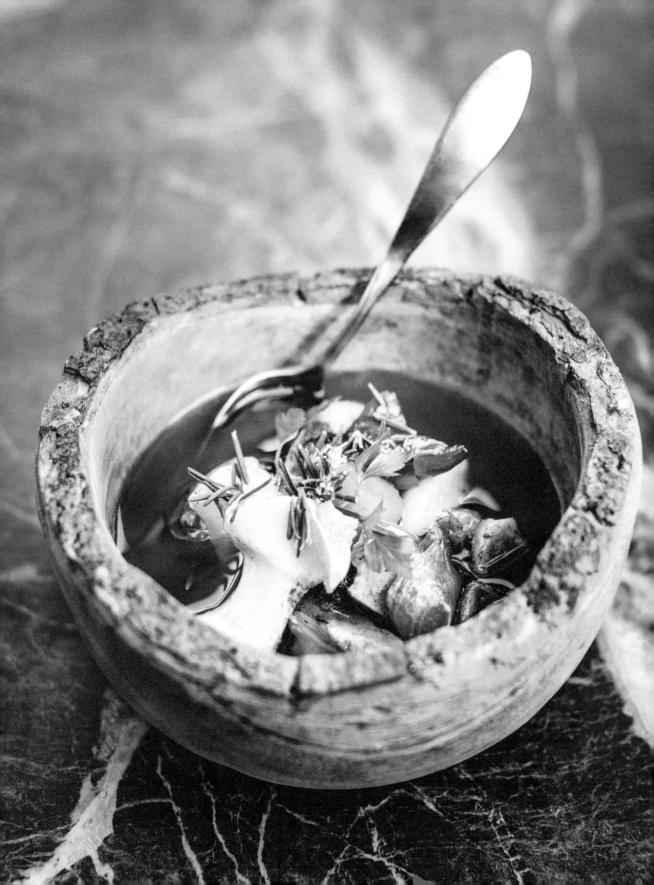

BONE BROTH

Serves: **2**

Time: **12-72 hours**

INGREDIENTS

1 kg beef, pork or chicken bones (can be combined)

4 carrots

4 celery stalks

1 chilli pepper

salt

ground pepper

2 bay leaves

3 litres water

fresh rosemary

UTENSILS

pot, knife

- Place the bones, salt, pepper, chilli pepper and bay leaves into a pot and fill with plenty of water.

- Cook over high heat for 5-10 minutes or until the water starts to boil.

- When the water starts to boil lower the heat to the lowest setting possible and cover the pot.

- Let the broth cook for at least 12 hours. Occasionally lift the lid and stir.

- The longer you let it cook, the stronger the flavour of the broth will be.

- 30 minutes before serving the broth, toss the carrots and chopped celery into the pot.

- Serve the broth in a bowl and garnish with a sprig of rosemary.

TIP: This broth is packed with collagen and other wonderful properties that will help to regenerate your skin and bones.

CLAMS WITH WHITE WINE

👤 Serves: **2**

⏱ Time: **15 minutes**

INGREDIENTS

400g fresh clams

handful coriander

4 cloves garlic

250 ml white wine

salt

extra virgin olive oil

UTENSILS

pan, knife

- Dice the garlic and soften in a frying pan with a little olive oil.

- Add the clams in and stir gently. Do this for 1 minute.

- Pour in the white wine and slowly stir. Stir in the salt and chopped coriander. Cook the clams until they open.

- After the last clam opens, remove from the heat and serve.

TIP: Don't overcook the clams or leave them over the heat for longer than necessary. They harden quickly and lose their texture and properties.

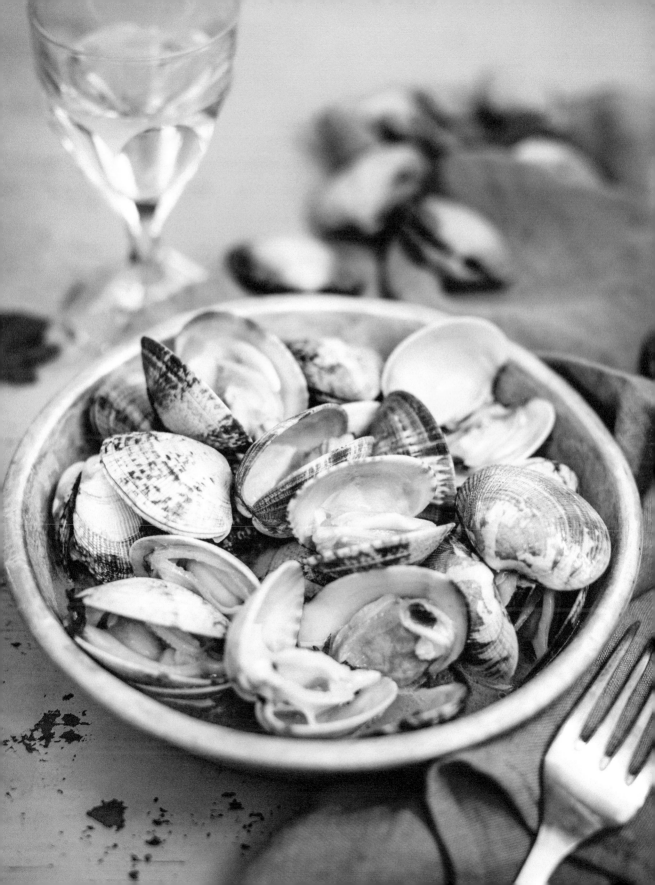

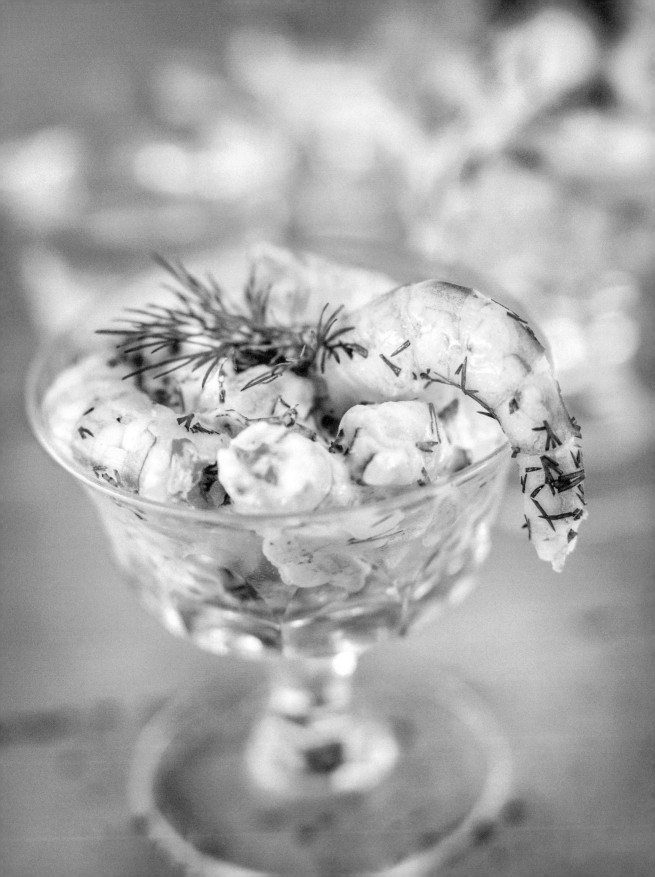

SKAGENRÖRA, SEAFOOD COCKTAIL NORDIC STYLE

👤 Serves: **2**

⏱ Time: **15 minutes**

INGREDIENTS

300g raw prawns

60 ml natural homemade mayonnaise (see page 240)

60 ml sour cream

60 ml lemon juice

32g dill

32g red onion

1 tsp Dijon mustard

salt

pepper

UTENSILS

pot, knife

- Cook the prawns for 5-10 minutes.

- Drain and let cool completely.

- Peel the prawns.

- Chop the dill and onion into fine pieces. The smaller the better.

- In a bowl, mix together the chopped onion, dill, mayo, sour cream, lemon juice, mustard and salt and pepper.

- Stir until all the ingredients are combined well and you have a uniform sauce.

- Add the completely cooled prawns into the sauce and mix well.

- Serve the skagenröra in a dish of your choosing and garnish with a sprig of dill.

TIP: Even though this recipe is super simple, it's chic. On special occasions you can pair it with some Cava or Champagne.

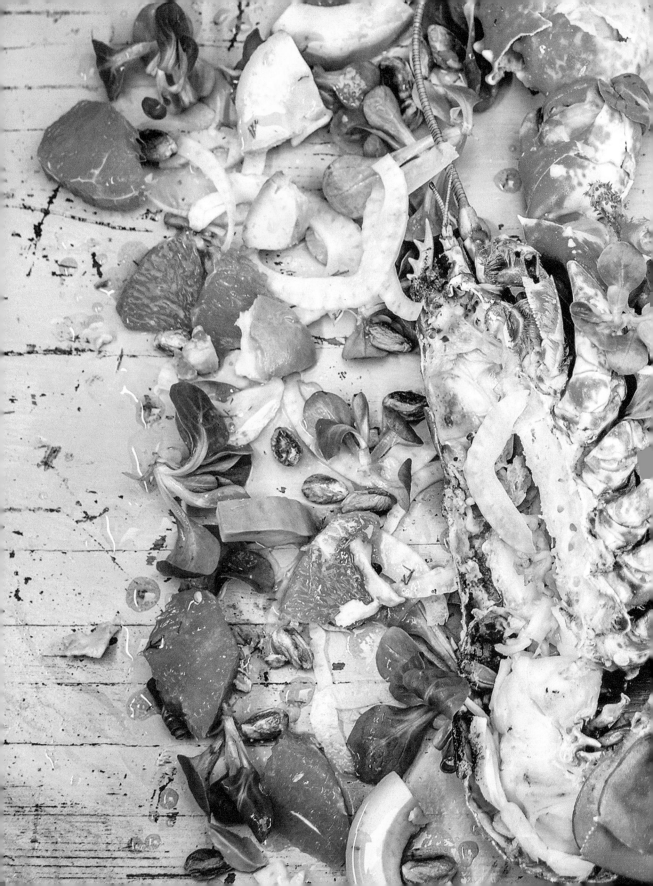

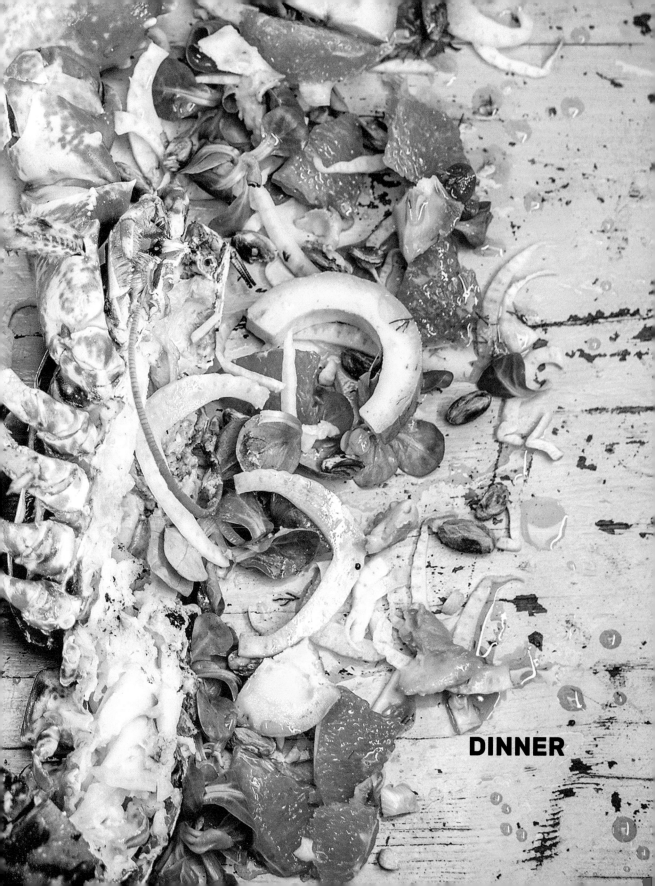

DINNER

SAUTEED DUCK BREAST WITH CURRY SAUCE AND PAK CHOI

Serves: **2**

Time: **25 minutes**

INGREDIENTS

400g duck breast

2 pak choi

200 ml curry sauce
(see page 245)

extra virgin olive oil

UTENSILS

pan, pot, knife

- Make square cuts on top of the duck breast.

- Drizzle some olive oil into your frying pan.

- Place the duck in the pan, skin side down.

- Cook over medium heat. About 10 minutes on the skin side and 5 minutes on the other side.

- In a pot, cook the pak choi with water and salt for 10 minutes.

- Remove the duck breast from the pan and let it rest for a few minutes before cutting it.

- Serve the duck breast on top of some curry sauce and place the pak choi on the side.

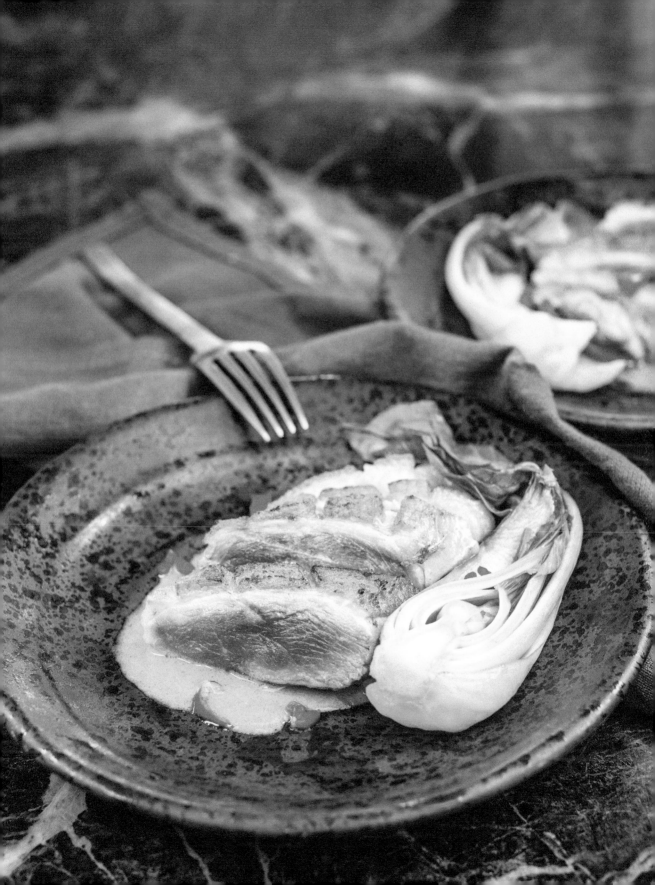

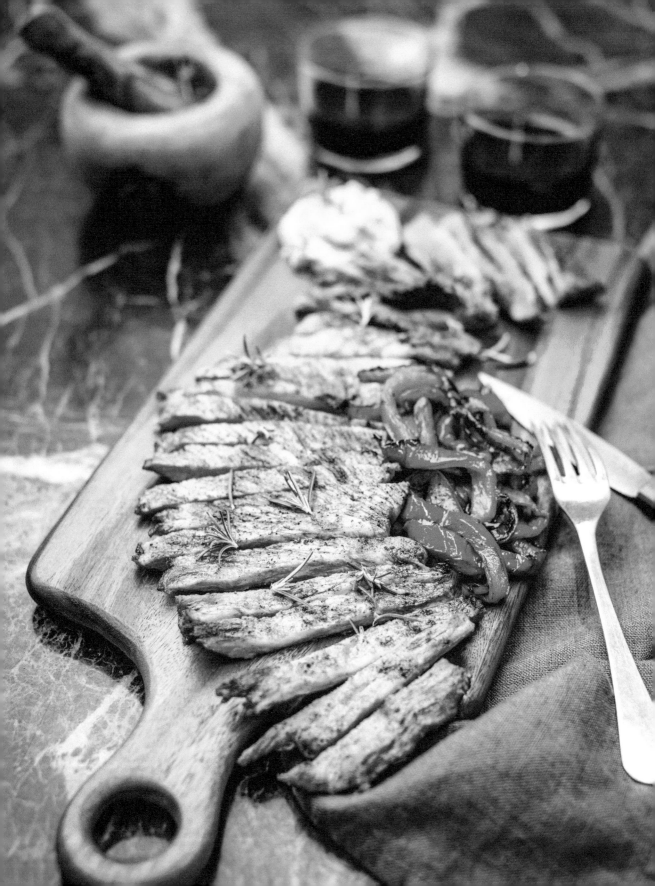

IBERIAN HAM WITH BABA GANUSH AND RED PEPPERS

 Serves: **2**

Time: **25 minutes**

INGREDIENTS

300g Spanish Iberian ham

1 red pepper

100g baba ganush
(see page 246)

flaked salt

½ handful fresh rosemary

UTENSILS

grill, knife

- First prepare the baba ganush. You can even do this the day before to save time.

- Make small cuts in the upper region of the ham.

- Place it on the grill and cook it for 10 minutes on each side over medium heat.

- Grill the red pepper at the same time.

- Make sure the pepper doesn't burn and that it cooks evenly.

- Remove the pepper and the Iberian ham from the grill. Then cut it into slices and sprinkle on the flaked salt.

- Serve the Iberian ham and grilled red pepper together with the baba ganush. Garnish with a fresh sprig of rosemary.

TIP: You can remove the skin from the red pepper if you wish or if it was accidentally overcooked.

SWEETBREAD BREADED IN BUCKWHEAT WITH BROCCOLI AND BACON

Serves: **2**

Time: **30 minutes**

INGREDIENTS

300g veal sweetbread

150g broccoli

100g buckwheat flour

100g bacon

32g chives

2 garlic cloves

2 tbsps butter

extra virgin olive oil

1 egg

UTENSILS

Pan, paper towel, bowl, knife

- Wash and chop the broccoli and garlic. Sauté in a pan with 2 tbsps of butter for 15 minutes over medium-low heat.

- Chop the bacon and place it in a separate pan. There is no need to add any oil or butter. Fry the bacon until it is crunchy.

- Cut the sweetbreads into 1cm pieces. Salt to taste.

- Beat the egg in a bowl and put the buckwheat in a separate bowl. Dip each piece of sweetbread in the egg first and then cover in buckwheat.

- Grease another frying pan with 4 tbsps of butter. Let the pan get hot and then fry the sweetbreads. Brown each side well. 5 minutes per side should be enough.

- If you feel the sweetbreads soaked up too much butter and are a bit greasy then place them on some paper towel after removing them from the pan.

- Serve the sweetbreads with some bacon on top and garnish them with some chopped chives. Accompany this with the broccoli.

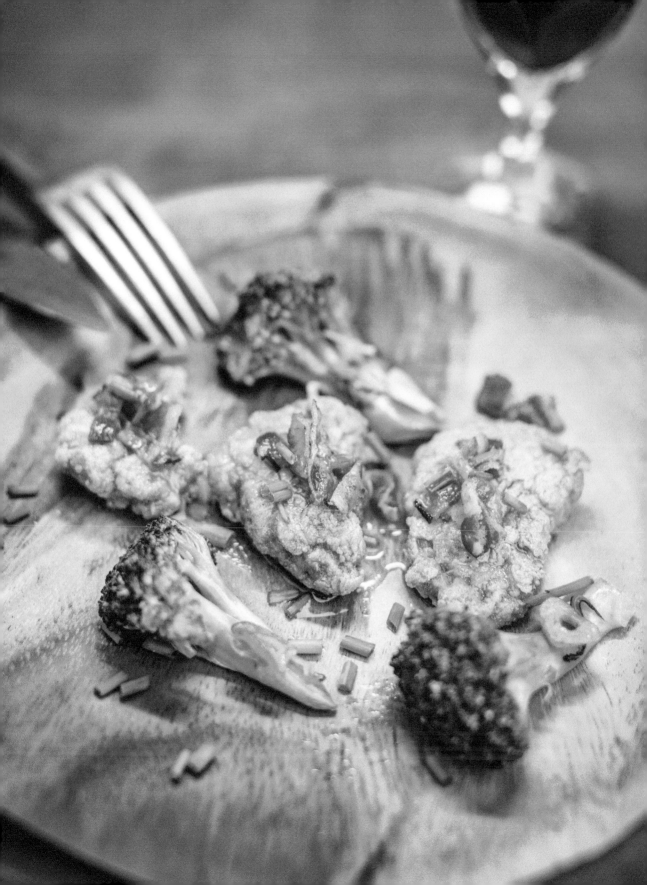

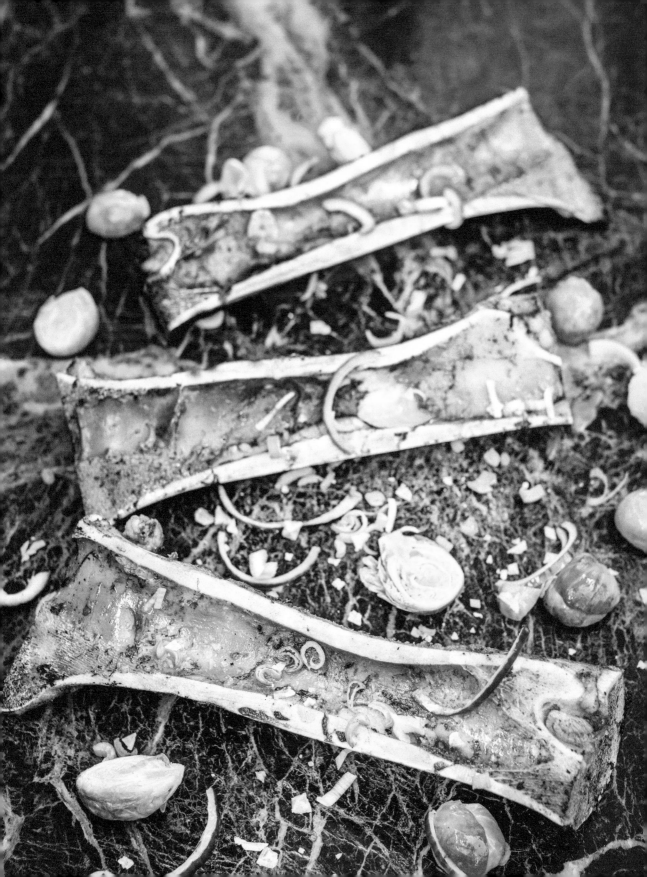

GRILLED VEAL MARROW WITH RED ONION AND BRUSSEL SPROUTS

Serves: **2**

Time: **30 minutes**

INGREDIENTS

800g veal shank bones

200g Brussels sprouts

1 red onion

32g chives

2 tbsps butter

salt and pepper

UTENSILS

grill, pan, knife

- Wash and chop the onion and Brussels sprouts.

- Melt the butter in a pan and sauté the Brussels sprouts with the onion until tender. Salt and pepper to taste.

- Season the bone with salt and pepper on the side with the marrow.

- Place the bones on the grill and cook them on the smooth side first for 15 minutes over medium heat.

- Turn the bones over and cook for another 10 minutes.

- Dice the chives.

- Serve the bone marrow with the onions and Brussels sprouts and sprinkle the chives over everything.

TIP: Be careful and make sure that the marrow doesn't burn or catch fire. If this happens, immediately remove the bones from the grill and turn down the flames.

SEARED VENISON WITH BÉARNAISE SAUCE

👤 Serves: **3**

⏱ Time: **30 minutes**

INGREDIENTS

400g venison sirloin

3 carrots

2 parsnips

coarse or flaked salt

100g béarnaise sauce
(see page 247)

UTENSILS

grill, knife

- Wash and cut the carrots and parsnips into strips. They should be on the large side but they don't all have to be exactly the same.

- Prepare the Béarnaise sauce and set aside.

- Cook the vegetables on the grill for 20 minutes on medium-low heat. Make sure to move them around so they don't burn.

- Remove the vegetables from the grill and set aside.

- Place the meat on the grill and cook for 5 minutes on each side.

- Once cooked, remove the meat from the grill and sprinkle some coarse flaked salt on top of the meat.

- Using the vegetables as a base, place the meat on top and finish the dish with the Béarnaise sauce.

TIP: Grill the meat to your liking. I prefer mine on the rarer side but feel free to cook yours longer.

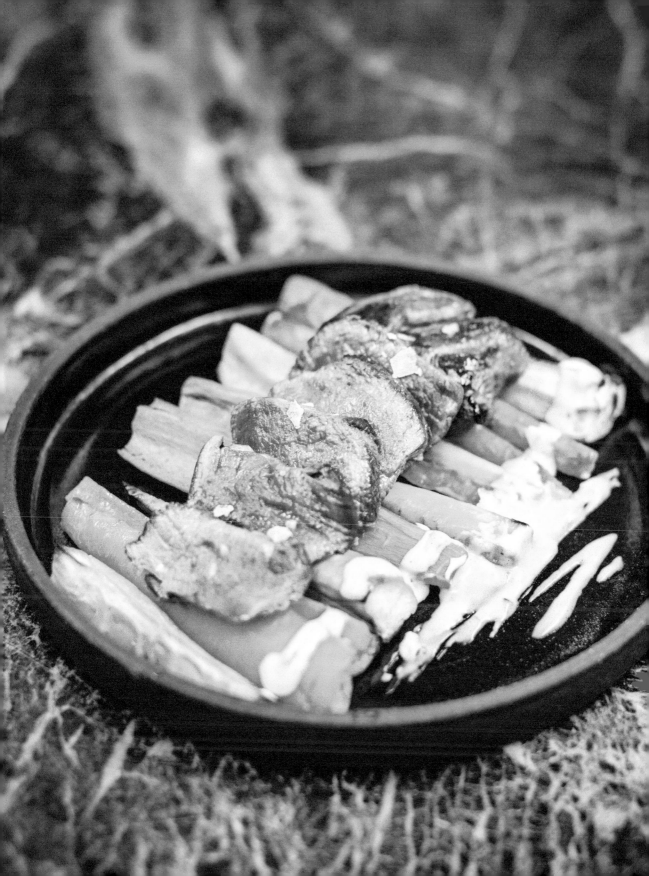

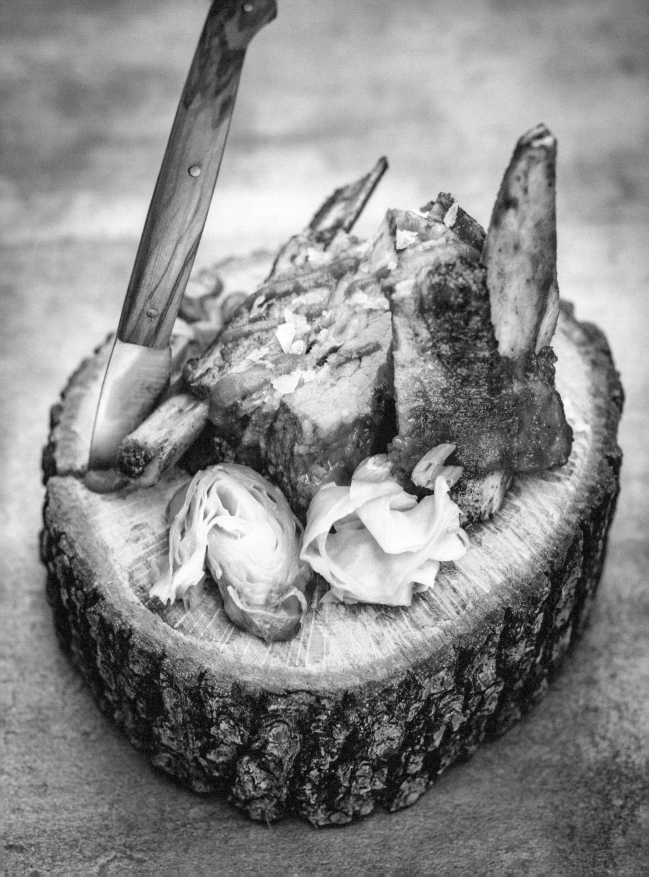

BARBECUE RIBS AND BRUSSELS SPROUTS

Serves: **2**

Time: **1 hour**

INGREDIENTS

500g beef ribs

4 Brussels sprouts

fresh chives

salt and pepper

barbecue sauce
(see page 241)

UTENSILS

pressure cooker, grill, knife

- Fill the pressure cooker with water three fingers deep.

- Place the ribs in the pressure cooker and cook on high heat for 45 minutes.

- Cook the sprouts in a separate pot with salted water for 10-15 minutes, then set aside.

- Remove the ribs from the pressure cooker when they are ready.

- Season the ribs with salt and pepper then brown them on the grill. Brush the barbecue sauce on the ribs and allow a crust to form.

- Centre the ribs on a plate and place the Brussels sprouts on the side. Drizzle a little barbecue sauce on top of the ribs and garnish with fresh chives.

TIP: Don't worry if you don't have a pressure cooker. Cook the ribs in a pot filled with water for about two hours.

PANCETTA WITH A CABBAGE SALAD

👤 Serves: **2**

⏱ Time: **90 minutes**

INGREDIENTS

400g pancetta

250g padrón peppers

200g red cabbage

3 carrots

100g homemade natural mayonnaise (see page 240)

extra virgin olive oil

salt and pepper

UTENSILS

pressure cooker, oven, pan, grater

- Place the pancetta in the pressure cooker and cook for 45 minutes.

- Preheat the oven to 175° C.

- Carefully remove the pancetta from the pressure cooker and place it on a baking sheet. Bake for 45 minutes or until the outer layer is golden brown and crispy.

- Drizzle some olive oil in a frying pan and fry the padrón pepper then set aside.

- Wash, grate and season the red cabbage and carrots.

- Add a little black pepper to the natural mayonnaise to give it a special touch.

- Mix the red cabbage and carrots in a bowl with the mayonnaise and pepper, forming a salad.

- Use the cabbage and carrot salad as the base of your dish and place the pancetta along with the padrón peppers on top. Drizzle a little more natural mayonnaise on one side of the plate for that professional touch.

TIP: If you don't have a pressure cooker use a normal pot filled with water and cook the pancetta for 1 hour and a half.

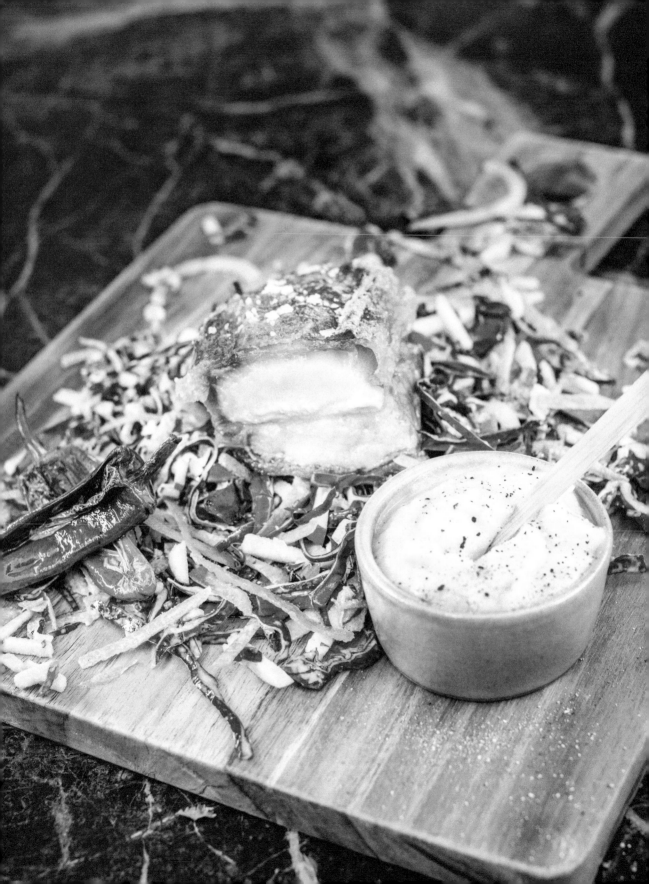

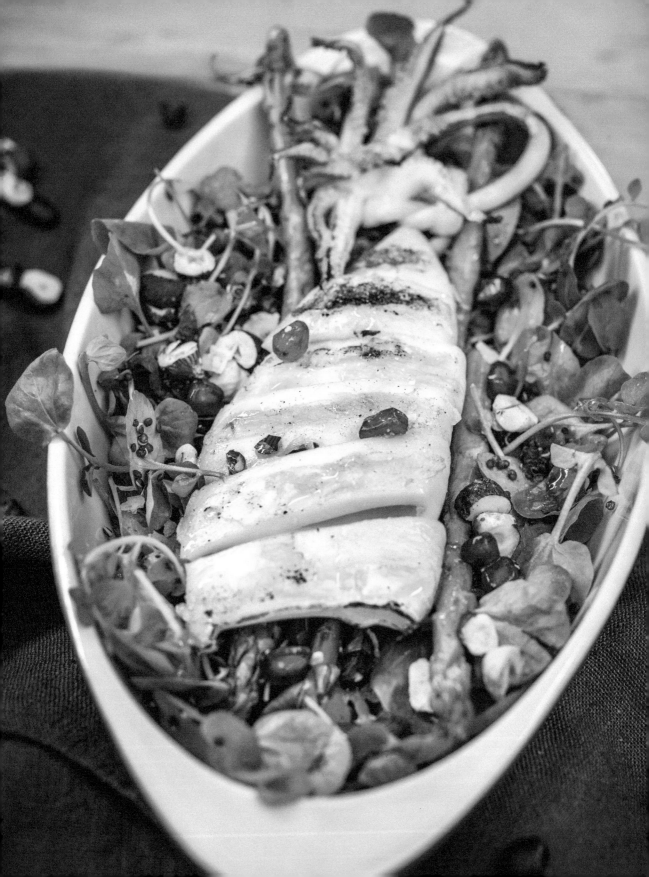

GRILLED SQUID WITH A FRESH SALAD

👤 Serves: **2**

⏱ Time: **15 minutes**

INGREDIENTS

1 large or 2 small squid

4 handfuls lamb's lettuce

½ pomegranate

64g unpeeled roasted hazelnuts

vinaigrette (see page 248)

UTENSILS

grill, knife

- Wash and clean the squid. Make small cuts to the upper region of the squid.

- Cook over medium heat on the grill for 5-10 minutes on both sides. The cooking time will depend on the size of the squid.

- In a bowl mix together the lamb's lettuce, pomegranate and hazelnuts to form a refreshing salad.

- Place the salad on the plate using it as a base for the squid. Dress your dish with the vinaigrette and there you have it.

KING PRAWN AND SEA BASS CEVICHE

⌂ Serves: **2**

⏱ Time: **20 minutes**

INGREDIENTS

150g raw sea bass

150g king prawn

handful coriander

100g papaya

½ mango

1 avocado

½ red onion

¼ chilli pepper

1 lime

natural mayonnaise
(see page 240)

UTENSILS

bowl, sharp knife

- Cut the sea bass into small chunks

- Squeeze half a lime into a bowl and season to taste. Marinate the sea bass in the lime mixture for at least 5-10 minutes.

- Chop the papaya, mango, avocado, red onion, coriander and chilli pepper into small pieces. Peel the prawns and chop them as well. Add the ingredients into the bowl and mix well.

- Squeeze in the other half of the lime and mix again.

- Serve up the ceviche with mayonnaise, and there you have it.

TIP: Serve this dish right away so that the fruit doesn't oxidise and the raw fish doesn't dry out or begin to smell bad.

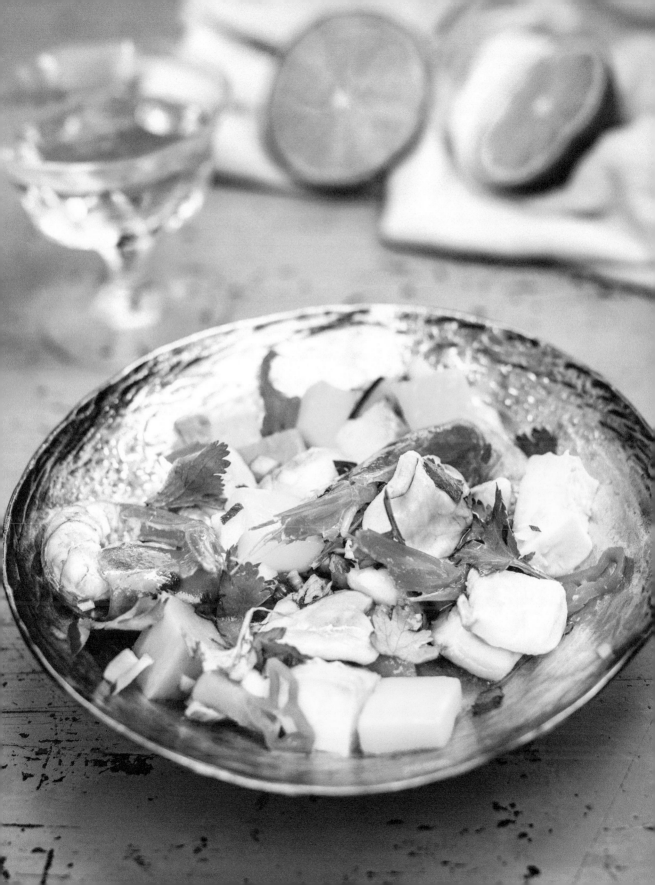

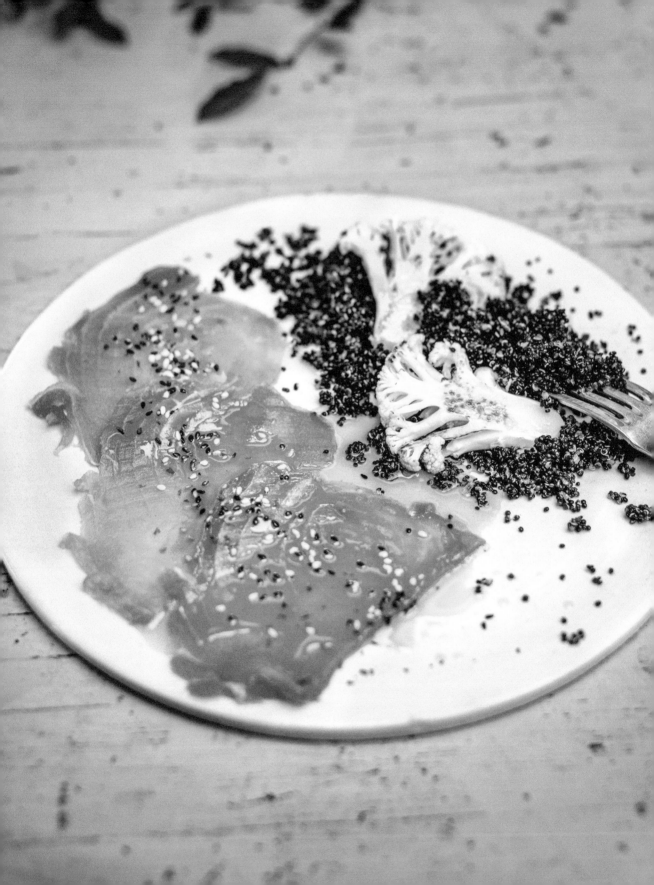

TUNA CARPACCIO WITH BLACK QUINOA AND FRIED CAULIFLOWER

👤 Serves: **2**

⏱ Time: **25 minutes**

INGREDIENTS

200g fresh bluefin tuna

125g black quinoa

500 ml water

200g cauliflower

½ handful sesame seeds

extra virgin olive oil

UTENSILS

pan, pot, very sharp knife

- Cook the quinoa in a pot with water and a little salt over high heat until the water starts to boil. Once the water boils, lower the heat and cook for another 15 minutes.

- Sauté the cauliflower in a pan with a little olive oil and salt.

- Cut the tuna into thin slices. Remember to always cut the tuna in the direction of the fish's veins.

- Plate all the ingredients as you wish and for that final touch drizzle some olive oil over the top and then sprinkle the sesame seeds all over the plate.

HAKE WITH A PARSNIP PURÉE AND DILL PESTO

👤 Serves: **2**

⏱ Time: **20 minutes**

INGREDIENTS

400g wild hake

6 parsnips

2 tbsps butter

handful dill

32g toasted pine nuts

32g parmesan cheese

32g cashews

1 garlic clove

2 radishes

salt

125 ml extra virgin olive oil

UTENSILS

blender or food processor,
frying pan, saucepan, knife

- Peel and cut the parsnips. Boil them in a pot filled with water for 15 minutes or until tender.

- Strain the water and then add butter and salt.

- Using a potato masher, mash the parsnips into a puree.

- In the food processor add the dill, pine nuts, cashews, garlic, parmesan, olive oil and a pinch of salt. Blend everything together well until you get a nice paste. If it is too pasty you can add more olive oil.

- Grease a frying pan with some olive oil and grill the fish; 3 minutes on each side is more than enough. Remember to always start on the side with the skin.

- Place some parsnip puree in the centre of your dish and spread some dill pesto over that. Then place the freshly grilled hake on top of that and garnish with a sprig of fresh dill. Add some thin slices of radish on the side and serve.

TIP: If you prefer classic basil pesto that works as well, just exchange the dill for fresh basil leaves.

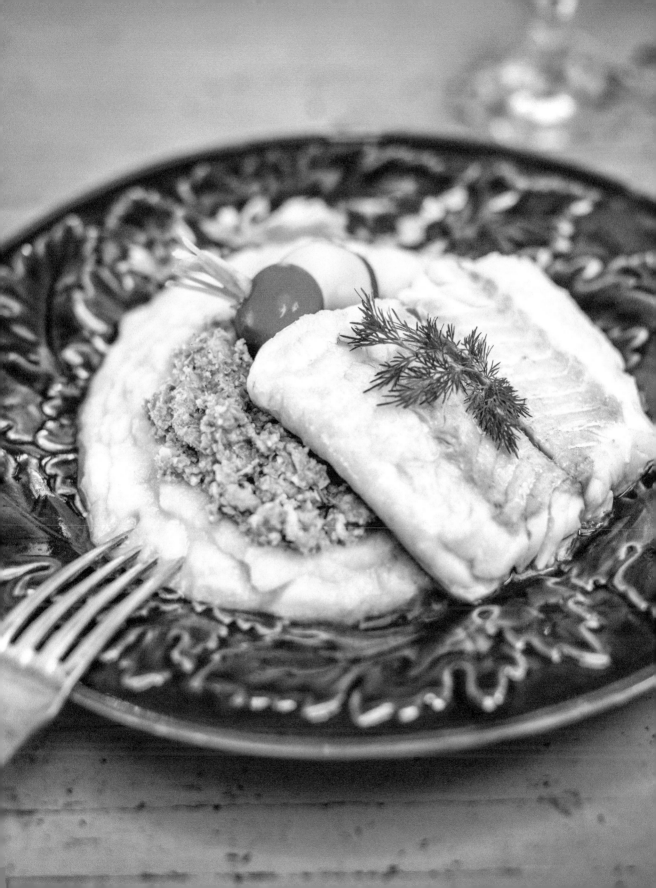

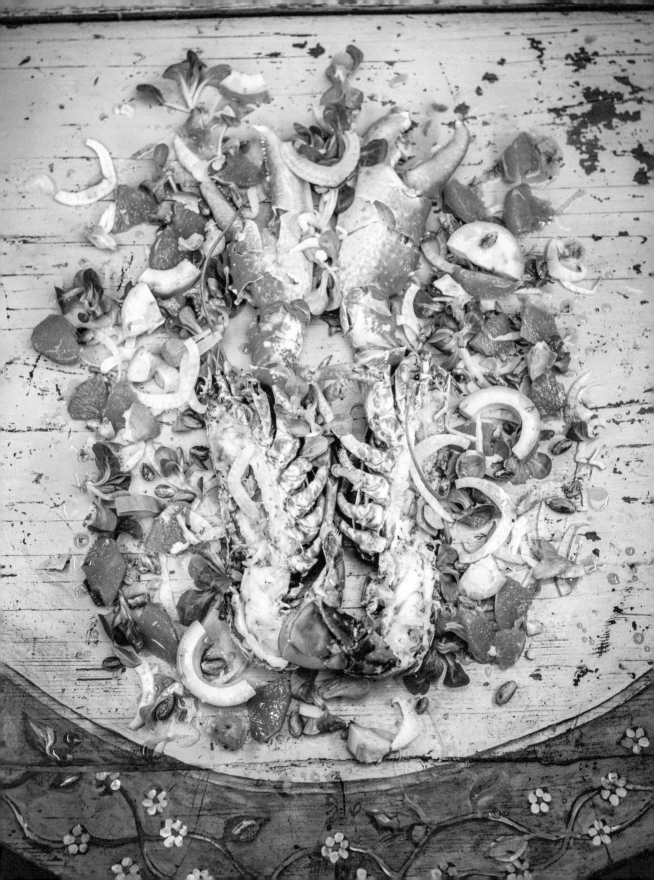

LOBSTER SALAD WITH A BALSAMIC VINAIGRETTE

👤 Serves: **2**

⏱ Time: **10 minutes**

INGREDIENTS

1 lobster

125g lamb's lettuce

1 bulb fennel

1 avocado

32g strawberries

64g peeled pistachios

vinaigrette (see page 248)

UTENSILS

grill, large sharp knife

- Using a large sharp knife cut the live lobster in half lengthwise. Next, with a cloth take the lobster by the head and insert the knife just where the body begins.

- Grill the lobster over medium heat for 10 minutes starting with the shell side first. Then flip it and cook it for another 5 minutes.

- Wash and chop the vegetables and fruit. Put together the salad by mixing the lamb's lettuce with the fennel, avocado, strawberries and pistachios. Use the vinaigrette as the dressing either on top of the salad or to the side.

- Place the lobster in the centre of the plate and scatter the salad around it.

SCALLOPS WITH A SWEET POTATO AND BEET PURÉE

👤 Serves: **2**

⏱ Time: **30 minutes**

INGREDIENTS

6 shelled scallops

200g beets

200g sweet potato

3 tbsp butter

100g snow peas

32g chives

salt

UTENSILS

pan, pot, knife, purée sieve

- Cook the beets and sweet potato in a pot for 20 minutes over medium-high heat. Salt to taste.

- Sauté the snow peas in butter for 2-5 minutes.

- Poke the sweet potatoes and beets with a knife. If the knife goes in smoothly, drain all the water and add 3 tablespoons of butter to the pot and mash everything together until you get a purée. Use a potato masher to get an even finer texture.

- Grease a clean pan with a little butter and heat it up. Griddle the scallops, they only need 30 seconds on each side.

- Time to assemble the scallops. Place some snow peas and purée on top of each scallop.

- Dice up some chives and sprinkle them over everything to give your dish that final touch.

TIP: If the scallops stick to the shell, remove them carefully and rinse them to remove any sand.

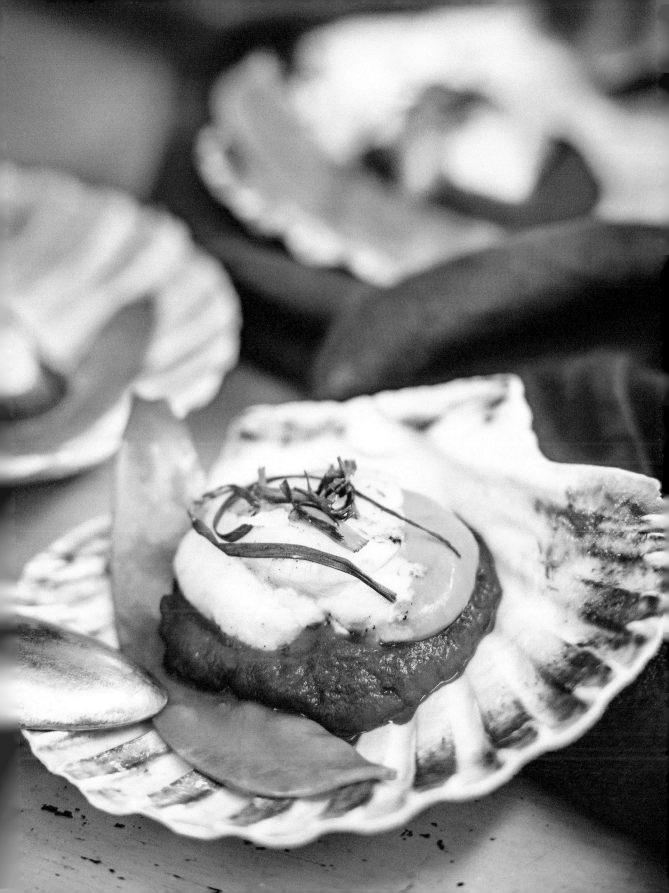

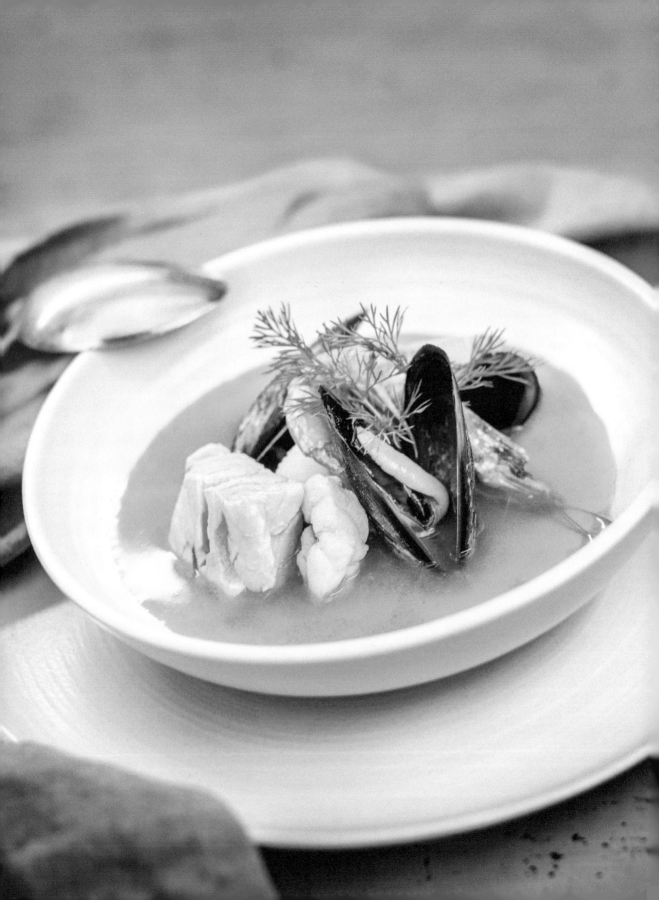

SEAFOOD BOUILLABAISSE

👤 Serves: **4**

⏱ Time: **3 hours**

INGREDIENTS

200g salmon

200g king prawns

200g monkfish

300g fresh mussels

500g fish bones (for the broth)

2g saffron

1 litre water

3 tbsps butter

½ handful dill

Salt

UTENSILS

pot, strainer, pan, knife

- In a large pot filled with salted water cook the fish bones for 2-3 hours. 10 minutes before finishing cooking the fish bones, add the saffron and butter.

- Peel the king prawns and clean the mussels well.

- Strain the broth and pour it into the pan.

- Cut the fish into cubes and put them in the broth. Add the prawns and mussels and let cook for 5 minutes.

- Serve the bouillabaisse and garnish it with a few sprigs of dill.

TIP: This dish should be served right away. For some added flavour add a little alioli sauce (made with crushed garlic and oil).

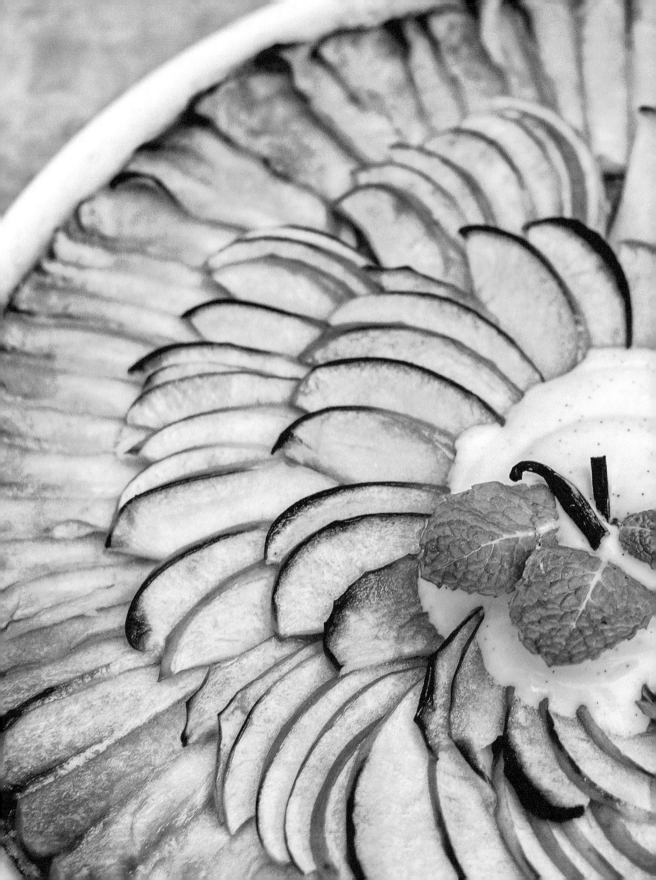

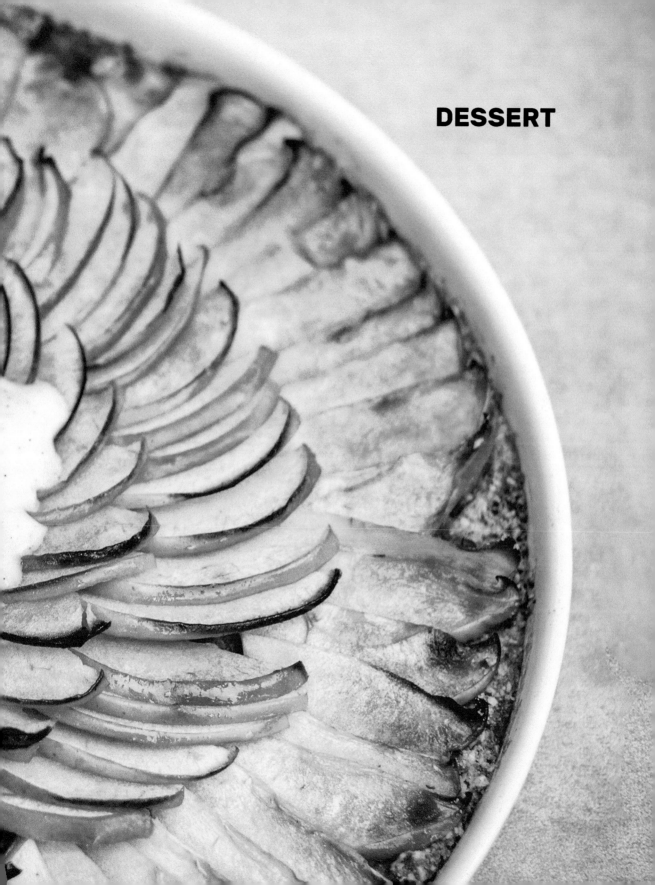

DESSERT

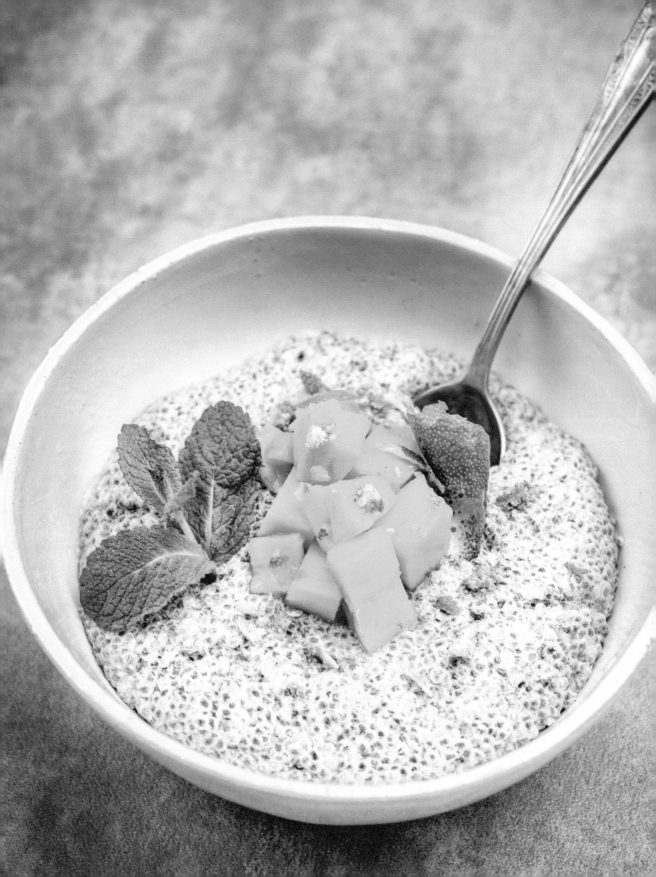

CHIA PUDDING

Serves: **2**

Time: **15 minutes + 4 hours**

INGREDIENTS

4 tbsps chia seeds

375 ml coconut milk

1 tsp raw honey

1 tsp vanilla bean paste or 1 vanilla pod

1 mango

1 lime

fresh mint

UTENSILS

bowl with lid, spoon, grater, knife

- In a bowl with a lid, mix together the chia seeds, coconut milk, honey and vanilla. Stir until everything is combined well.

- Cover and let sit for 2 minutes.

- Uncover and stir again. Then cover it back up and place it in the fridge to chill for at least 4 hours.

- Remove the pudding from the fridge and serve in a bowl.

- Slice some diced mango to put on top of the pudding along with some lime zest. Garnish with a few fresh mint leaves.

TIP: If you'd like to enjoy this delicious pudding for breakfast, make it the night before so it can set in the fridge while you sleep. Also, if you like a more intense flavour, you can add extra lime juice.

APPLE TART

Serves: **6-8**

Time: **30 minutes**

INGREDIENTS

4 apples

64g butter, melted

64g buckwheat

125g almond flour

1 egg yolk

1 tbsp coconut sugar

125g crème fraîche

1 tsp raw organic honey

½ vanilla pod

2-3 fresh mint leaves

UTENSILS

spatula, oven, pie dish,
knife

- Preheat oven to 225° C.

- Melt the butter and mix it in with the buckwheat, almond flour, egg yolk and coconut sugar.

- Grease the pie dish with butter and place the dough in as the base. Using a spatula flatten the dough and create an even base.

- Cut the apples into thin slices and place them on top of the dough in a circular shape.

- Put the tart in the oven and bake for 30 minutes or until the apples have turned a golden-brown colour.

- While the tart is baking get started on the crème fraîche. Mix together the créme fraîche honey and vanilla.

- Remove the tart from the oven and let cool for a few minutes.

- Pour the cream on top of the tart and garnish with some mint leaves.

TIP: To extract the vanilla beans from the pod, spread out the pod and hold it by the edges. With a knife, cut the pod lengthwise. Then with the back of the knife, press lightly until the entire inside of the vanilla pod is removed.

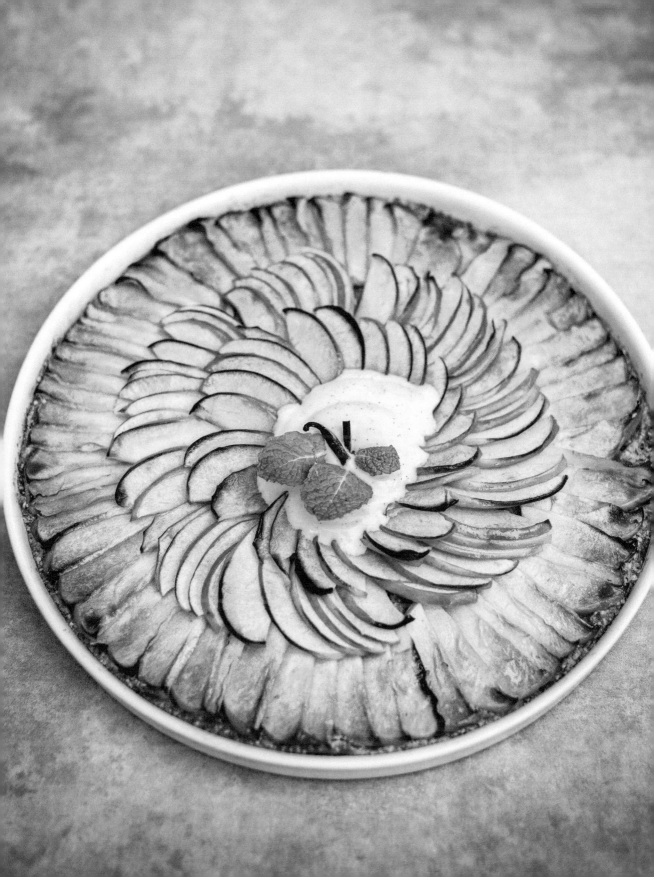

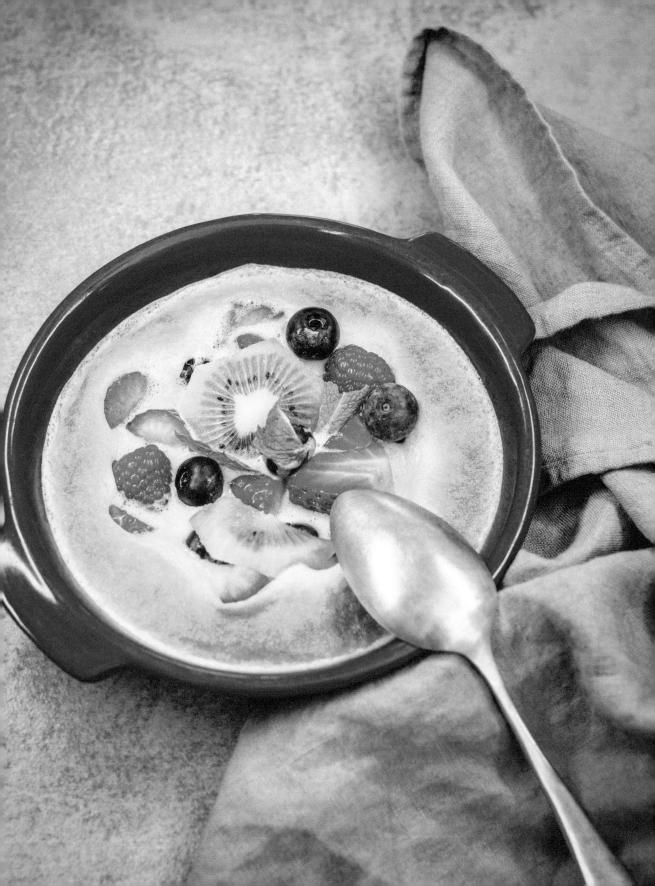

FRUIT ZABAGLIONE

👤 Serves: **2**

🕐 Time: **15 minutes**

INGREDIENTS

6 egg yolks

2 tbsps coconut sugar

1 tbsp sherry wine

pinch of salt

1 kiwi

1 strawberry

4 raspberries

4 blueberries

mint leaf

UTENSILS

whisk, double boiler, 2
individual baking tins,
knife

- Preheat oven to 250° C.

- Separate egg yolks from whites

- In a bowl add the egg yolks to the sugar, and wine
with a pinch of salt.

- Place the bowl over a pot of boiling water (double
boiler). Whisk vigorously for 5-8 minutes.

- When the mixture becomes creamy, remove it from
the heat.

- Divide the cream equally into two individual
baking tins.

- Cut the fruit and divide it between the two tins.

- Place both baking tins in the oven and bake for 5
minutes.

- Remove from the oven when they have turned a
nice golden-brown colour.

- Garnish with some fresh pieces of fruit and mint
leaves.

TIP: Customise this dish with your favourite fruits and add as much as you'd like!

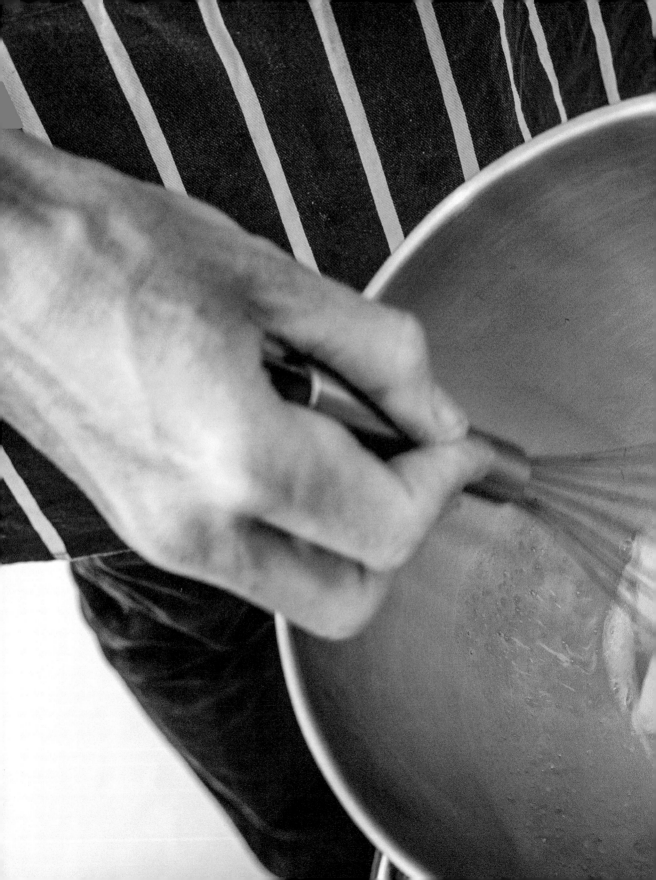

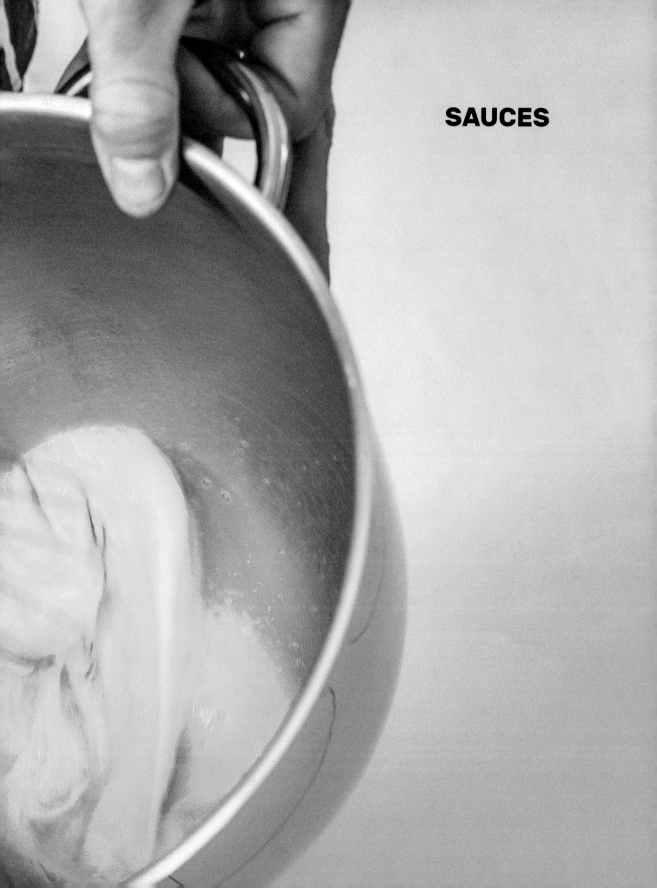

SAUCES

HOLLANDAISE SAUCE

Serves: **4**

Time: **30 minutes**

INGREDIENTS

½ lemon

150g ghee or clarified butter

4 egg yolks

pinch of salt

UTENSILS

whisk, pot

- Melt 150g butter in a saucepan and let cook for 20 minutes.

- Remove all the foam that forms on top of the surface with a ladle. Do not stir the butter while it is cooking.

- Separate 4 eggs yolks from their whites. Then whisk them together in a bowl.

- When the eggs have started to whip, begin adding the ghee/clarified butter. Make sure to skim off the whey and not add it in to the eggs. Do this process slowly as you constantly whip the eggs.

- After you've fully blended in the ghee, add the juice from half a lemon and a pinch of salt.

- Finish blending all the ingredients and serve with your dish.

TIP: If you already have some ghee prepared then just add it in, in its liquid form. This sauce is ideal with eggs, fish and seafood.

TOMATO SAUCE

👤 Serves: **4**

⏱ Time: **2 hours**

INGREDIENTS

6 vine tomatoes or equivalent in cherry tomatoes

2 tbsps organic butter

1 garlic clove, minced

4 basil leaves

salt and pepper

250 ml natural tomato puree

UTENSILS

pot/saucepan, blender or food processor, knife

- Melt the butter in a saucepan and brown the minced garlic, making sure that it doesn't burn.

- Add the diced tomatoes and sauté them for 5 minutes or until they begin to break and release their natural juices.

- Next add the puree and salt and pepper to taste. Stir everything together.

- Cover the pot and let the sauce cook for another hour and a half over low heat.

- If the sauce becomes too thick, you can add ½ glass of water.

- When the sauce is finished, top it off with some fresh basil leaves.

TIP: This sauce can be chunky as it is here but if you prefer something smoother just run the tomatoes through a blender or food processor before you cook them. This sauce is the perfect base for a Bolognese or ratatouille. You can also make a wonderful shakshuka with this natural tomato sauce.

MAYONNAISE

👤 Serves: **4**

⏱ Time: **20 minutes**

INGREDIENTS

1 organic egg

500 ml extra virgin olive oil

2 tbsps Dijon mustard

1 tsp salt

UTENSILS

hand blender or whisk

- Add the egg, mustard and salt to a bowl and whisk together vigorously.

- Slowly and steadily pour the olive oil into the mixture.

- Don't stop whisking until the sauce emulsifies and you get the creamy smooth texture you want. Be careful not to whisk it for too long as this can cut the texture.

- Once finished, place your homemade mayo in an airtight jar and store it in the fridge.

TIP: A chef's trick is to place the bowl on a damp kitchen towel so that the bowl doesn't move as you whisk. Also, this frees up your other hand so that you can add the oil more consistently. If you accidentally cut the mayonnaise, beat another egg in a separate bowl and add it in little by little until the mayonnaise emulsifies again. This sauce is great with eggs, vegetables, fish, fried foods or as a salad dressing. It is also a wonderful spread for fajitas and hamburgers.

BARBECUE SAUCE

👤 Serves: **4**

⏱ Time: **40 minutes**

INGREDIENTS

2 tbsps butter or ghee

1 small onion

3 garlic cloves

3 tbsps tomato paste

¼ tsp cayenne pepper

1 tsp Dijon mustard

1 tsp sweet paprika

½ tsp salt

60 ml white vinegar

60 ml water

3 tbsps raw honey

UTENSILS

pot /saucepan, hand
mixer or whisk, knife

- Melt the ghee or butter in a saucepan and brown the chopped onion and garlic for 5 minutes over medium-high heat.

- Next place all the ingredients together with the ghee mixture in a blender and blend for 2-3 minutes until you get a uniform sauce

- Pour the sauce into a pot and cook over low heat for 40 minutes, stirring occasionally with the whisk so that nothing sticks to the bottom of the pot.

- Once the sauce becomes creamy, remove it from the heat and let rest for 10 minutes.

- Either use it directly or store it in a glass jar that has an airtight seal and place it in the fridge. It will stay fresh for up to a week.

TIP: This sauce is wonderful for pork dishes, wings and fried foods. You can even spread it on top of your hamburger to give it an American touch.

HOMEMADE GUACAMOLE

👤 Serves: **4**

⏱ Time: **10 minutes**

INGREDIENTS

3 medium ripe avocados

1 lime

64g chopped coriander

½ red onion

salt to taste

UTENSILS

large bowl, knife, mortar
(optional)

- Open the avocados and remove the seed from the centre then remove the outer skin. Cut the avocado into chunks in order to make them easier to smash.

- Chop up the onion and coriander into very small pieces. Add them and the avocado into a large bowl.

- Squeeze the lime juice over everything.

- Mash all the ingredients using a fork or mortar.

- Add some salt in little by little tasting as you go until you get the perfect combination for you.

TIP: If you are going to store any leftover guacamole, cover the stone with some cling wrap and place it in the container. It will stay fresh longer this way. Guacamole is great with chicken, fish, seafood and fried foods. And of course, you can't forget to use it in your favourite Mexican dish!

TZATZIKI SAUCE

Serves: **4**

Time: **30 minutes + 2 hours**

INGREDIENTS

500 ml plain Greek yogurt

2 cucumbers

2 garlic cloves

½ lemon

4 tbsps extra virgin olive oil

coarse salt and pepper

½ handful chopped dill or mint

UTENSILS

mortar, grater, strainer, whisk, colander

- Mince the garlic and add it to the mortar along with some coarse salt. Crush it up well until a paste forms. Place the paste in a separate bowl.

- Next, peel the cucumbers and cut them in half. With the help of a spoon, remove all the seeds. Grate the cucumbers and sprinkle them with salt.

- Place the grated cucumbers in a colander and let them drain and release as much water as possible.

- In the same bowl where you placed the garlic paste, add the yogurt, olive oil, finely chopped dill and the juice from half a lemon. Stir everything well until you get an evenly distributed and uniform texture.

- Store the mixture in the fridge while you continue to let the cucumber drain.

- After the grated cucumber is dry, take the mixture from the fridge and add the cucumber. Mix well.

- Then place it back in the refrigerator and let sit for at least a couple of hours before serving.

TIP: This yogurt sauce is ideal for salads, meats, vegetables, fish and seafood. Don't forget this special sauce when you make your moussaka. It will definitely raise the level of your dish.

BÉCHAMEL

Serves: **4**

Time: **15 minutes**

INGREDIENTS

112g butter

1 tbsp tapioca flour

1 tbsp buckwheat flour

500 ml whole milk
or almond milk
(see page 249)

125g grated semi-cured
cheese

pinch nutmeg

salt and pepper to taste

UTENSILS

pot, sieve or strainer,
whisk

- Sift the tapioca flour and buckwheat flour through a sieve or thin strainer.

- Melt the butter in a pot. After the butter has melted add the flour and beat with a whisk for 2-3 minutes over medium heat.

- When bubbles start to form add the milk little by little. Do not stop beating the mixture with the whisk until all the milk is integrated and it begins to curdle.

- Next, add the salt, pepper and nutmeg.

- Lastly, throw in the cheese and stir everything until it has melted into the sauce. Remove from the heat and let rest.

TIP: If you can have milk use it. However, if you are lactose intolerant or simply don't like milk then use the almond milk. Use this French sauce for gratin, to enrich creams, or to mix with vegetables or to make delicious croquettes. You can even top off moussaka with a béchamel gratin for an even tastier dish.

CURRY SAUCE

Serves: **2**

Time: **15 minutes**

INGREDIENTS

250 ml water

4 lemongrass stems

4 kaffir lime leaves

1 tbsp organic red curry paste

400 ml coconut milk (for cooking)

salt and pepper

UTENSILS

pot, whisk

- In a clean pot, boil 250ml water with the lemongrass stems, lime leaves and red curry paste for 5 minutes.

- Whisk everything until the paste has completely dissolved.

- Remove the pot from the heat and season to taste.

- Gradually whisk in the coconut milk until combined well.

- Put the pot back on the heat for 10 more minutes on low heat.

- Let sit for a couple of minutes then remove the lemongrass stems and lime leave before serving.

TIP: Make your Indian style dishes more traditional and complete with this sauce.

BABA GANUSH

👤 Serves: **4**

⏱ Time: **50 minutes**

INGREDIENTS

3 aubergines

extra virgin olive oil

1 large or 2 small cloves garlic

1 lime

pinch salt

1 tsp powdered cumin

2 tbsp tahini or sesame paste

UTENSILS

grill, mortar, knife

- Grill the whole aubergines for 40 minutes over medium heat. Move them around so they cook evenly on all sides.

- Remove the aubergines from the grill and set aside to cool.

- Crush the garlic in the mortar until a paste forms.

- Use a knife to cut the aubergines in half. Remove the flesh from the interior with the help of a spoon and place it into the mortar.

- Add the lime juice along with the tahini, cumin, salt and olive oil. Keep mashing everything until you get a paste-like puree.

TIP: If you don't have a grill just put the aubergines in the oven for 40 minutes at 175° C. This sauce is great as an Arabian style dip/spread or to serve as a starter with meats.

BÉARNAISE SAUCE

👤 Serves: **2**

🕐 Time: **30 minutes**

INGREDIENTS

2 egg yolks

250g ghee or butter

10 ml tarragon vinegar

10 ml white wine

½ handful tarragon/
estragon

black peppercorns

2 shallots

salt and pepper

UTENSILS

pot, whisk, strainer, large
glass or metal bowl

- Dice the shallots as small and thin as possible. Add them into the saucepan along with the white wine, vinegar and a few black peppercorns (to taste).

- Cook over medium heat until the liquids have reduced by half.

- Remove the pot from the heat and strain the mixture then set aside and let cool.

- In a double boiler, mix the egg yolks together with the previously strained mixture.

- Whisk vigorously and gradually add the ghee (or melted butter).

- When the sauce is finished, add the tarragon and season to taste.

TIP: This French sauce is great to pair with meats but it can also be used with fish, vegetables and eggs.

VINAIGRETTE

👤 Serves: **2**

⏱ Time: **5 minutes**

INGREDIENTS

2 tbsps olive oil

1 tbsp balsamic vinegar

½ tbsp raw honey

salt

UTENSILS

Whisk

- Add the olive oil, balsamic vinegar, honey and salt into a bowl.
- Whisk together vigorously until everything is evenly combined leaving you with a uniform dressing.

TIP: This is the go-to dressing for all your salads. You can also add a drizzle of this vinaigrette to your stir-fries to give them a special touch.

ALMOND MILK

Serves: **2**

Time: **8 hours + 20 minutes**

INGREDIENTS

125g raw, peeled almonds

1 litre water

UTENSILS

blender or food processor, gauze or fine mesh

- Cover the almonds in 500 ml water and let them soak for at least 8 hours.

- Drain the almonds and place them in the blender with another 500 ml clean water.

- You can add any sweetener of your choice.

- Blend the mixture for 1-2 minutes on full power or until all the almonds have been completely crushed.

- In a deep mixing bowl, place some gauze or mesh. Next, pour in the mixture.

- Using your hands. Squeeze the gauze until the milk is strained.

- There should be only a paste or some almond flour left inside the gauze after it is strained.

- Store the milk in the refrigerator in an airtight container for up to 4 days.

TIP: For sweetness I recommend adding 1 teaspoon of raw honey.

RECIPE INDEX

BREAKFAST

138   ASPARAGUS AND SHIITAKE MUSHROOM OMELETTE

141   EGGS FLORENTINE WITH SPINACH AND HOLLANDAISE SAUCE

142   AÇAI BOWL WITH KIWI, BANANA, BLUEBERRIES AND GRATED COCONUT 142

145   NATURAL WAFFLES

NATURAL SMOOTHIES

148   BANANA AND COCOA SMOOTHIE

151   GREEN SMOOTHIE

152   WILD STRAWBERRY AND HAZELNUT SMOOTHIE

155   GINGER VITAMIN SMOOTHIE

APPETISERS, SNACKS AND BREADS

158   CRUNCHY SEED CRACKERS

161   CHIA AND WALNUT BREAD

162   DATE, NUTS AND CHIA BARS

165   FOIE GRAS CANAPES WITH CARAMELISED ONION

LUNCH

169   SHAKSHUKA

170   ROASTED AUBERGINE SALAD WITH GOAT'S CHEESE

173   COURGETTI WITH TOMATOES AND BASIL

174   KALE AND SPINACH CREAM SOUP WITH PARMESAN CRISPS

177   NAPOLITANA PIZZA

178   CRÈME FRAÎCHE PIZZA WITH SALMON EGGS AND RED ONION

181   PASSION FRUIT AND IBERIAN HAM PIZZA

182   ROASTED PINEAPPLE WITH TUNA BELLY

185   VENISON TARTARE WITH SEEDED CRISPBREAD

186   MINI HAMBURGERS

189   CHICKEN WITH SWEET POTATO FAJITAS

190   MOUSSAKA WITH TZATZIKI

193   BONE BROTH

194   CLAMS WITH WHITE WINE

197   SKAGENRÖRA, SEAFOOD COCKTAIL NORDIC STYLE

DINNER

200   SAUTEED DUCK BREAST WITH CURRY SAUCE AND PAK CHOI

203   IBERIAN HAM WITH BABA GANUSH AND RED PEPPERS

204   SWEETBREAD BREADED IN BUCKWHEAT WITH BROCCOLI AND BACON

207   GRILLED VEAL MARROW WITH RED ONION AND BRUSSEL SPROUTS

208   SEARED VENISON WITH BÉARNAISE SAUCE

211   BARBECUE RIBS AND BRUSSELS SPROUTS

212   PANCETTA WITH A CABBAGE SALAD

215   GRILLED SQUID WITH A FRESH SALAD

216   KING PRAWN AND SEA BASS CEVICHE

219   TUNA CARPACCIO WITH BLACK QUINOA AND FRIED CAULIFLOWER

220   HAKE WITH PARSNIP PURÉE AND DILL PESTO

223   LOBSTER SALAD WITH BALSAMIC VINAIGRETTE

224   SCALLOPS WITH A SWEET POTATO AND BEET PURÉE

227   BOUILLABAISSE

DESSERTS

231   CHIA PUDDING

232   APPLE TART

235   FRUIT ZABAGLIONE

SAUCES

238   HOLLANDAISE SAUCE

239   TOMATO SAUCE

240   MAYONNAISE

241   BARBECUE SAUCE

242   HOMEMADE GUACAMOLE

243   TZATZIKI SAUCE

244   BÉCHAMEL

245   CURRY SAUCE

246   BABA GANUSH

247   BÉARNAISE SAUCE

248   VINAIGRETTE

249   ALMOND MILK

References

(All links correct at time of printing)

Ahrens, E.H., Hirsch, J., Insull, W., Tsaltas, T.T., Blomstrand, R., Peterson, M.L. (1957) Dietary Control of Serum Lipids in Relation to Atherosclerosis. *JAMA*, 164 (17): 1905–1911.

Bazzano, L., Hu, T., Reynolds, K., Yao, L., Bunol, C., Liu, Y., Chen, C., Klag, M., Whelton, P. and He, J. (2014) Effects of Low-Carbohydrate and Low-Fat Diets. *Ann Intern Med.* 161 (5): 309–18.

CDC (2020) National Health and Nutrition Examination Survey. [online] Available at: https://www.cdc.gov/nchs/nhanes/index.htm

Eurostat (2019) Over half of adults in the EU are overweight. [online] Available at: https://ec.europa.eu/eurostat/web/products-eurostat-news/-/ddn-20210721-2

Eurostat (2021) Cardiovascular Diseases Statistics. [online] Available at: https://ec.europa.eu/eurostat/statistics-explained/index.php?title=Cardiovascular_diseases_statistics#Deaths_from_cardiovascular_diseases

Herrera-Covarrubias, D., Coria-Avila, G.A., Fernández-Pomares, C., Aranda-Abreu, G.E., Manzo Denes, J., & Hernández, M.E. (2015) Obesity as a risk factor in the development of cancer. *Rev. perú. med. exp. salud publica*, 32 (4)

Lustig, R., (2012) Pure White and Deadly. *Tapa blanda* (International edition), 25, December.

Lustig, R. et al. (2016) Isocaloric fructose restriction and metabolic improvement in children with obesity and metabolic syndrome. *Obesity (Silver Spring, Md.)* 24 (2): 453–60.

Ma, Y., Yang, Y., Wang, F., Zhang, P., Shi, C., Zou, Y., Qin, H. (2013) Obesity and risk of colorectal cancer: a systematic review of prospective studies. *PLoS One.* 8 (1): e53916.

McNamara, D.J. (2015) The Big Fat Surprise: Why Butter, Meat and Cheese Belong in a Healthy Diet, by Nina Teicholz. Reviewed by DJ McNamara. *The American Journal of Clinical Nutrition*, 102 (1): 232.

Natruly Blog (2021) *Home – Natruly Blog.* [online] Available at: https://blog.natruly.com/en/.

New York Times. (1986) *F.D.A. Report Splits on Effects of Sugar.* [online] Available at: https://www.nytimes.com/1986/10/02/garden/fda-report-splits-on-effects-of-sugar.html.

NHS Digital (2019) Health Survey for England. [online] Available at: https://digital.nhs.uk/data-and-information/publications/statistical/health-survey-for-england/2019

O'Connor A. (2016) How the Sugar Industry Shifted Blame to Fat. *New York Times*, Sept. 12, 2016. [online] Available at: https://www.nytimes.com/2016/09/13/well/eat/how-the-sugar-industry-shifted-blame-to-fat.html.

OECD (2020) Health at a Glance: Europe 2020: State of Health in the EU Cycle. [online] Available at: https://www.oecd-ilibrary.org/

Public Health England (2020) Sugar reduction: progress report, 2015 to 2019. [online] Available at: https://www.gov.uk/government/publications/sugar-reduction-report-on-progress-between-2015-and-2019

Rieser, S., Michaelis IV, O., Putney, J., Hallfrisch, J. (1975) Effect of Sucrose Feeding on the Intestinal Transport of Sugars in Two Strains of Rats. *The Journal of Nutrition*, 105 (7): 894–905.

Science Watch (2010) *Interview with Lewis Cantley, Harvard Medical School.* November 2010. [online] Available at: http://archive.sciencewatch.com/inter/aut/2010/10-nov/10novCant/.

Select Committee on Nutrition and Human Needs (1977) Dietary Goals for the United States. [online] Available at: https://naldc.nal.usda.gov/download/1759572/PDF. Oecd-ilibrary.org. 2021.

Serra-Majem, L. (2010) Nutrición Comunitaria y sostenibilidad: concepto y evidencias. *Rec Esp Nutr* Comunicatio, 16 (1): 35-40.

Seven Countries Study (n.d.) *The Seven Countries Study - The first epidemiological nutrition study, since 1958.* [online] Available at: https://www.sevencountriesstudy.com.

Stare, F. (1975) Sugar in the diet of man. In: Bourne, GH editor. *World Rev Nutr Diet.* 22: 237–326.

Taheri, S., Lin, L., Austin, D., Young, T., Mignot, E. (2004) Short sleep duration is associated with reduced leptin, elevated ghrelin, and increased body mass index. *PLoS medicine*, 1 (3): e62.

Taubes, G. (2002) *What if It's All Been a Big Fat Lie?* [online] Available at: https://www.nytimes.com/2002/07/07/magazine/what-if-it-s-all-been-a-big-fat-lie.html.

Taubes, G. (2011). *Is Sugar Toxic?* [online] Available at: https://www.nytimes.com/2011/04/17/magazine/mag-17Sugar-t.html.

Taubes, G. (2016) *The Case Against Sugar.* New York: Alfred A. Knopf.

Taubes, G. and Couzens, C. (2012) *Big Sugar's sweet little lies.* Mother Jones. November 2012 Issue. [online] Available at: https://www.motherjones.com/environment/2012/10/sugar-industry-lies-campaign.

TIME.com. (1984). *TIME Magazine Cover: Cholesterol,* Mar. 26, 1984. [online] Available at: http://content.time.com/time/covers/0,16641,19840326,00.html.

WHO (2015) *Guideline: sugars intake for adults and children.* [online] Available at: https://www.who.int/publications/i/item/9789241549028.

Yang, Q., Zhang, Z., Gregg, E.W., Flanders, W.D., Merritt, R., Hu, F.B. (2014) Added Sugar Intake and Cardiovascular Diseases Mortality Among US Adults. *JAMA Intern Med.*, 174 (4): 516–524.

Yudkin, J. (1972) *Pure, White and Deadly.* New York: P.H. Wyden

Yudkin, J. (1972) *Sweet and Dangerous.* New York: P.H. Wyden